Becoming a Fighter: Yoga, Music & Story Telling

Magic Happens at the Museum of Reincarnation

First Edition

ISBN: 979-8-218-06407-5

Registration Number: TXu002216109

In each story, any references to historical events, real people, or real places are used fictitiously. Names, characters, and places are products of the author's imagination.

Printed in the United States of America.

First printing edition 2022.

[1]**"Ezekiel saw the wheel, Way up in the middle of the air**

The big wheel runs by faith, And the little wheel runs by the grace of God

There is a wheel in a wheel."

"William L. Dawson"

چو شادی بکاهد بکاهد روان   خرد گردد اندر میان ناتوان

" فردوسی "

Translation:

When happiness is gone, the psyche is incapable, Then wisdom becomes weak and feeble

When the fountains of happiness begin to flow, Then the psyche and the wisdom begin to grow

[2] *"Ferdowsi"*

"Hold fast to dreams. For when dreams die, life is a broken wing bird that cannot fly."

"Langston Hughes"

---

[1] "Ezekiel Saw the Wheel" is a folk song written by William L. Dawson.
[2] The Shahnameh ("The Book of Kings") is a long epic poem written by the Persian poet Ferdowsi between c. 977 and 1010 CE and is the national epic of Iran. Consisting of some 50,000 "distiches".

Acknowledgements

Thank you to my family who supported me all my life and contributed to the cultivation of my growth and development. A special thanks to my brother who is an inspirational guru and instrumental in the creation of the photographs, the audio files, and the whole package. With you everything is possible and without you, life is a "broken wing bird that cannot fly."

Table of Contents

<u>Preface</u>

To quote Dr. Martin Luther King, Jr. "I Have a Dream Speech, I have a dream that is rooted in the American dream, that all men are created equal." There are obstacles, there are barriers, but there are no limits. Understanding yourself is the first step. Remember the longest journey begins with the first step, and that first step determines the direction your journey will take.

This book is an entertainment delicacy that includes layers of storytelling, music, a museum, and yoga. These layers of languages and ways of knowing blend together revealing self-knowledge of the mind and body. You will experience the story of a young woman, Natalia, who grows into adulthood and becomes a warrior woman. Listen and pat your feet, and dance as the story of Natalia unfolds from a teenager's first party to an adult finding justice in the city.

This book was born out of my passion to integrate education with yoga and music, specifically the integration of storytelling, song, music, the wisdom of famous people, deepening cultural understanding, and the yoga. The blending of storytelling and music is a part of human traditions that echo across the millennia. It is also the basis of the language of music that attracts, motivates, and from which young people learn. The Museum of Reincarnation is a museum in which the individuals meet famous people who share the wisdom of the ages. In the virtual museum we meet famous men and women in history. The portraits are alive, and learners meet Martin Luther King, Jr. Ludwig von Beethoven, Marie Curie, Hatshepsut, George Washington, Florence Nightingale, and Albert Einstein. Young people are reincarnated as they absorb the spirit, wisdom, and knowledge of these great leaders. Yoga practices inform the embodied self that enjoys music and storytelling.

The audiences for this book are open-minded people who have a passion for development of the self by embracing new experiences such as short stories, music, wisdom words, deepening cultural understanding and yoga. At the end of this book, you will have experienced different ways of understanding the world.

There are seven chapters in this book. This introductory chapter (Chapter 1) is constructed to give you a general picture of the structure of all the chapters that are to follow. Chapters 2 to 7 tell the story of Natalia and her growth and development. Chapter 2 is about Natalia's first teenage party. Chapter 3 is about Natalia as an eighteen-year-old girl pretending she and her friend are superstars going to a party. In Chapter 4, Natalia falls in love with a young man she meets in the park, Chapter 5 is about Natalia waiting for her boyfriend to come home from a trip. Chapter 6 is entitled, Liar, and Natalia discovers that her love has been deceiving her. Chapter 7 is about Natalia becoming a warrior and finding justice after having her heart broken and her money taken.

It is necessary to mention that all the lyrics, audios, videos, and the website are original and created out of my passion for integrating different ways of understanding the world. I hope you enjoy it!

Elham Zandvakili

Chapter 1: Introductory Chapter

Section 1: Short Story: The EZ Way

"The EZ Way"

Once upon a time Dr. EZ decided to make her dream come true and integrate her passion for teaching language with music, yoga, and storytelling. Her goal is to encourage English language learners to feel as if they have the strength of the mountains. They are strong as mountains, and they can reach the sky. They are not like sands in the desert moving from one place to another. To accomplish this, she recognized that she needed to encourage the students to build their inner strength. So, one day she sat and wrote down some of her ideas as an introduction to her book. Here is what came to her mind:

"Students will learn best when they feel their inner strengths and are grounded and balanced. When they have achieved this, they are ready for learning. So, clap your hands, pat your feet! Dr. EZ is in the house. It is time to learn English in an easy way. Let us get out of the old classroom, let us find peace through yoga and then go where the music is exciting. Sing, dance, and rock to the music. Feel the strength and the power of the flow of energy as you move to the music. This is a distinguished model. It is time to sing, dance, and learn English together. We can learn English forever."

Section 2: Song and Lyrics: The EZ Way

"The EZ Way"

It's time to connect and integrate

Language, Culture with Yoga and Music

with a chic unique technique

Dr.EZ has made it sweet and very easy

Believe me her method is fun and very breezy

Language learning through the music

Through a story which is so rhythmic

Hey, you English language learners

Let's go beyond (the class) let's go further

Let's go learn English

This new model is distinguished

and cannot be extinguished

It's Time to sing, dance and learn together

Today, tomorrow maybe forever

Do not ever panic, it is so romantic

We are all on fire, we are full of desire

Be as determined and strong as a mountain

Listen to streams of energy from your fountain

Section 3: Museum of Reincarnation: Martin Luther King Jr.

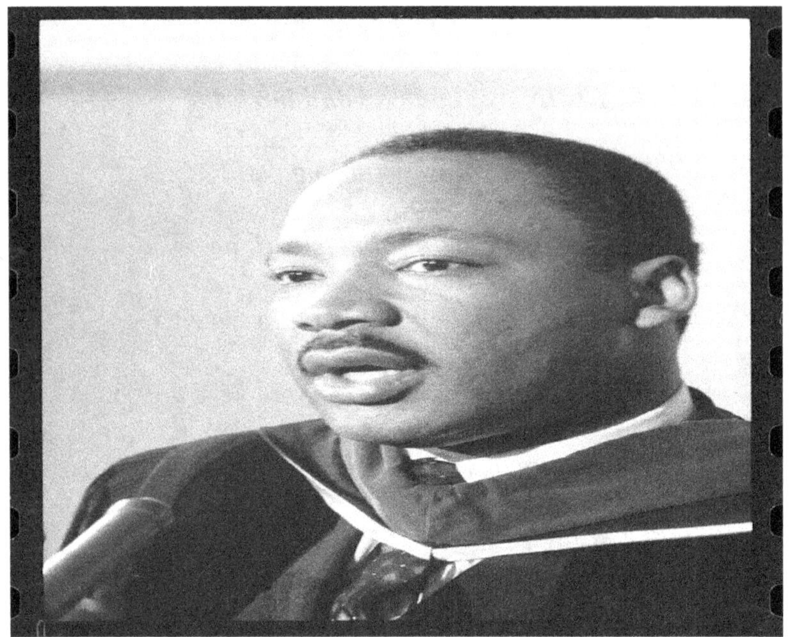

Leffler, W. K., (1965) *Martin Luther King*

The biography part of the museum (Visit website to listen)

Visiting the museum (Visit website to watch and listen)

Museum Transcripts

a. Biography

Martin Luther King, Jr. (1929-1968) was an African American Christian [3]civil rights

[4]leader who was the face of the civil rights movement. His [5]vision and philosophy of [6]non-

violence was a great counterpoint to the violence and threats from those who [7]advocated [8]racial

---

[3] Civil rights include freedom, equality in law and in employment, and the right to vote.
[4] a person in control of a group, country, or situation
[5] Idea
[6] a situation in which someone avoids fighting or using physical force, especially when trying to make political change
[7] supported
[8] connected with someone's race

[9]segregation. His career began with his leadership of the Montgomery, Alabama, bus [10]boycott to [11]protest segregated seats on buses. Under his influence, buses, restaurants, and schools were desegregated. Dr. Kings' vision of civil rights evolved beyond racial segregation to confront the evils of economic [12]inequality. He was [13]assassinated in Memphis, Tenn, while organizing a poor people's march for [14]economic opportunity and equity in 1968 ("Martin Luther King Jr.," n.d.; Carson, C. (2001); Wikipedia contributors, 2022).

b. Paraphrased Quotations

Schools have two goals: to teach skills and techniques and to teach values and culture. Techniques belong to the material world, and values and cultures belong to the spiritual world. What matters is the spiritual world. Culture is all the good things that people value in their daily lives. I used to worry about integrating different cultures together. Today, I am not worried anymore. Now integration is the solution and not the problem. Will you be a part of culture that has made the world a better place to live? I still believe that pure truth and love are the solutions. Through nonviolence, peace is possible in the world. Nonviolence is the unique way beyond the darkness to the light. And beyond the light is where dreams come true. According to John 1:5 NLT: "The light shines in the darkness, and the darkness can never extinguish it." I have desires for non-violence, world peace, and a lack of poverty. Ultimately a distinguished nation is a compassionate nation. No individual or nation can be great if it is not worried about others. No, no, we are not satisfied, and we will not be satisfied until justice rolls down like waters and righteousness like a mighty stream. Let the rhythmic sound of freedom rings from the mighty

---

[9] the policy of keeping one group of people apart from another and treating them differently, especially because of race, sex, or religion

[10] to refuse to buy a product or take part in an activity as a way of expressing strong disapproval

[11] a strong complaint

[12] unfairness

[13] was killed

[14] relating to money

mountains. (123 Of the Most Powerful Martin Luther King Jr. Quotes Ever, Hannah Hutyra, 2019).

Section 4: Deepening our Cultural Understanding: "Immigrants in the Music Industry"

"Immigrants in the Music Industry" in the USA

With the help of immigrants, American music is loved around the world. [15]Slave songs and [16]gospels from the Caribbean, Africa, and the Bahamas changed into the blues (sad songs), [17]hip hop, and [18]R&B. We watch famous people on Dancing with the Stars performing salsa dance to the sound of Latino musical instruments. Country music is known as an American genre, with deep roots in the European immigrant musical traditions that were brought to the Appalachian region (Ideal Immigration, 2019).

There are many immigrants who have become famous musicians, such as Rihanna.

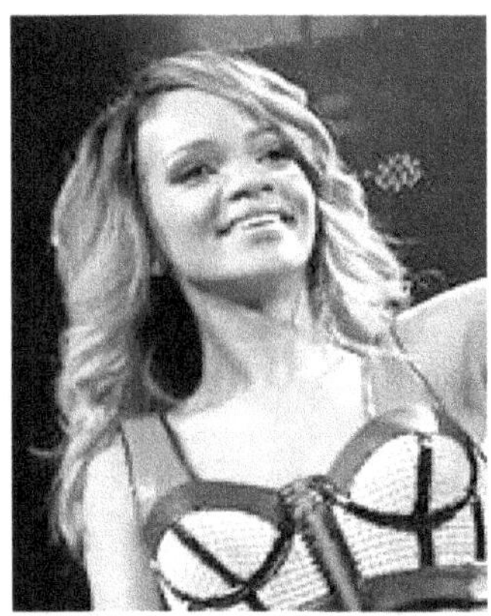

Pop star Rihanna was born in Saint Michael Parish, Barbados. After moving to the United States in 2004, she signed with Def Jam Recordings, starting her music career. (Newsday.com Staff, 2017); Not only did she bring a different taste of pop music to America but also, she recently [19]donated $5 million to help fight

---

[15] a person who is legally owned by someone else and must work for that person
[16] A music genre that originated during African American slavery
[17] a type of popular music in which the words are spoken rather than sung and the subject of the songs is often politics or society
[18] a type of popular music, originally by African American artists, that can have features of soul, jazz, funk, and hip-hop
[19] to give money or goods to help a person or organization

the [20]coronavirus. She is 32 years old, and she is the richest female singer in the world (Ellasar, 2020).

Immigrants are the source of change, inspiration, and new directions in popular music. These newcomers to America bring something new to the American musical experience. Their contributions continue to give new life, purpose, and meaning to popular music

Section 5: Yoga Posture: Mountain

A Rationale

"Yoga is one of the world's oldest traditions for seeking wisdom and truth." (Kripalu Manual, 2019). When you practice breathing and yoga, you free yourself to feel, to know, to relax, to enjoy, and to free yourself of doubts, anxieties, and pressures from your past. Through yoga, the negative emotions of anxiety, fear, and loneliness disappear from the school settings in which students learn English. Through yoga, you can look deeper inside yourself, and "Looking deeper gives you more options" (Carroll, 2019). Yoga without intention and self-awareness is exercise. Always set an intention when you start your yoga practice to be able to be aware and understand your thoughts (Meta-cognition), and your emotions (Meta- affection). Understanding the self includes knowing your thoughts and your emotions. When you monitor and control your thoughts and emotions, this leads you to understand your thoughts and emotions better ("Intra-personal Intelligence", Gardner, 1983), and consequently, you are able to fully engage and understand your relations with others ("Interpersonal Intelligence", Gardner,1983).

Each chapter in this book includes a main picture of a yoga posture (Asana) which is followed by the story of the mythology of that posture. Then a connection is made between the

---

[20] a type of virus that includes the SARS virus

posture and the short story. Next comes a yogic breathing (Pranayama) and warm-up exercise, and lastly, we have the posture steps accompanied by precautionary health notes. Avoid the postures if you have any doubts about your health, uncontrolled high or low blood pressure, or recent injuries to any affected areas.

The poem below includes the name of all the postures used in this book. The names are underlined so that you will be aware of the names.

🎧 Intro Poem to Yoga (Visit website to listen)

Be as determined and strong as a <u>mountain</u>

Listen to all the streams of your fountain

Imagine the big sky with a <u>half moon</u>

You are going to shine and complete the other half soon

Dream big, fly high like an <u>eagle</u>

Don't doubt your inner beauty, your inner regal

Sit on the glorious <u>chair</u> of your life

Don't be afraid of challenge and strife

Be as patient and as generous as a <u>tree</u>

Don't say, me and me, turn it to we

Don't be hesitant, you can break all the walls all the barriers

Be proud, be victorious, you are the <u>warrior,</u> you are the <u>warrior</u>

Yoga Posture: Mountain (Asana: Tadasana)
Tada: mountain; Asana: posture

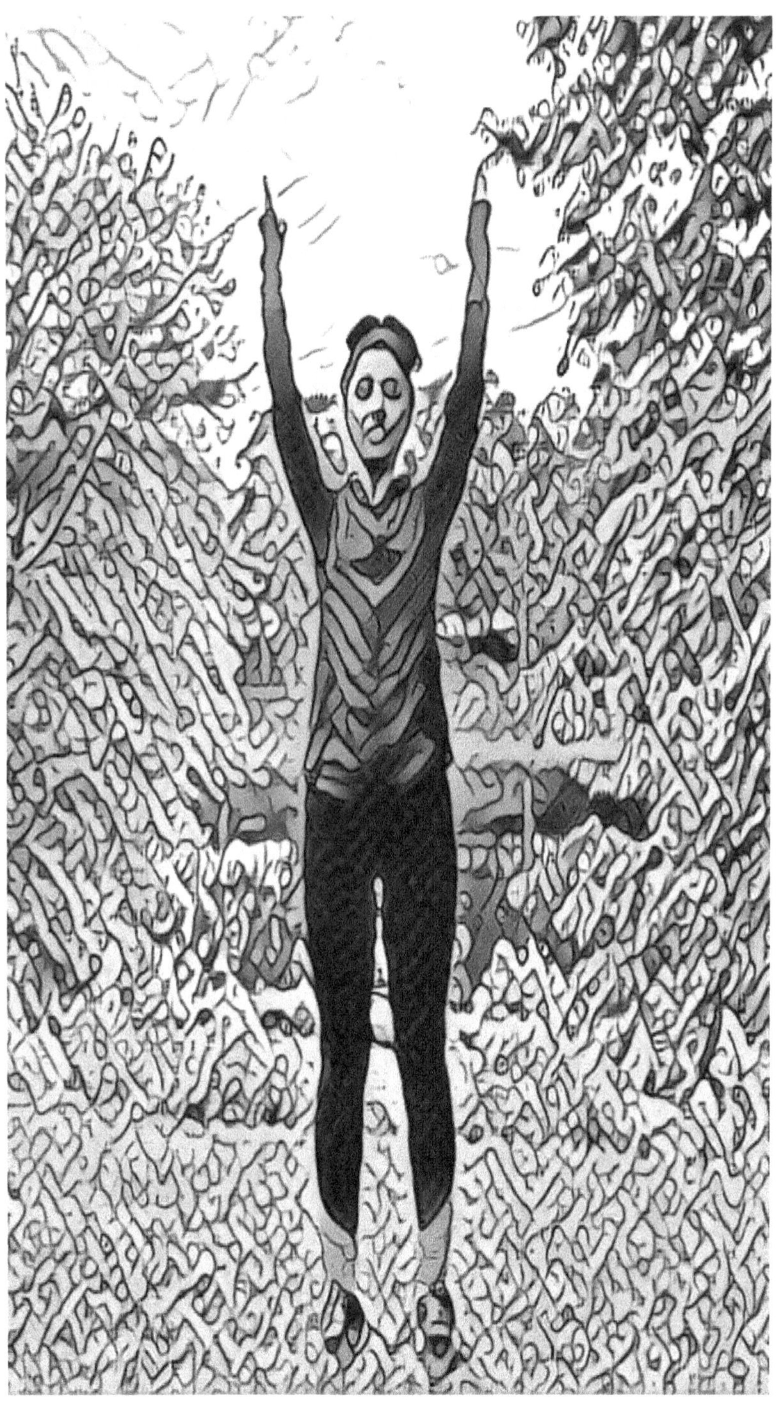

Stay strong as a mountain, no matter if the earthquakes of life shake you and make you want to collapse. Always remember you are a mountain!

Mythology of Tadasana

Tadasana is the mountain pose and the foundation for all standing postures. According to Kaivalya (2016), this pose "promotes the stillness, strength, relaxed power, and stability we associate with mountains." When you are inclined to feel grounded and balanced, you can imagine yourself *as* the mountain- standing tall, steady, and expansive (McGinley, 2017). The mountain symbolizes the rise toward the goal one wants to gain. Mountains are the home of the Gods and "are comparable to the sources of wisdom from which knowledge radiates in all directions, like rivers that flow from the mountain to nourish the land. So, approach the mountain freely and openly" (Radha, 2006). The mountain pose also symbolizes the flow of the energy throughout the body from the heaven to the earth. Energy flows through the body down the spine and anchors itself in the earth.

The holiness of the mountain and its position as a place of the saints is also reflected in the mysterious and beautiful stories of the [21]Shahnameh and [22]Alborz Mountain range (Dadvar & Rouzbahani, 2016).

Connecting the content of the lesson and the posture

1- The student must feel the strength and the power of being a mountain.

2- Feel the flow of knowledge and energy through your body.

3- Feel the streams and fountains of language, music, critical thinking, storytelling, and yoga.

---

[21] The Shahnameh is a long epic poem written by the Persian poet Ferdowsi between c. 977 and 1010 CE and is the national epic of Iran.
[22] The Alborz Mountain range in northern Iran stretches from the border of Azerbaijan along the western and entire southern coast of the Caspian Sea.

Cautionary notes

Do not hold the posture for a long period of time if you have any heart or circulatory issues, high or low blood pressure.

Yogic Breathing: Dirgha Pranayama

Meaning: Prana: air; life force; Yama: to restrain or hold back

Potential effects

Enhancement of complete and full breathing, decreasing stress and tension while calming the mind and the body, helping the lungs remain healthy by increasing the oxygen flow to the blood, it massages the abdominal organs, facilitating digestion, preparing you for a better learning experience. Breathing is the key to learning. Through breathing you are breaking down the emotional barriers to learning. Stop for a minute and remember how important breathing is.

Breathing Steps (Visit website to listen)

1- Sit up straight with your shoulders back and down with relaxed abdominals. Relax the face, close your mouth, and place your hands on your belly. Breathe into your belly and feel it expand like a balloon. Repeat a few times.

2- Now, put your hands to the sides of your rib cage and breathe into them, feeling the rib cage expand, and repeat a few times.

3- Put your fingertips on your upper chest. Breathe into it and feel your hands lifting. Repeat a few times.

4-Now, place your hands on your thighs with your palms facing up and make a complete inhalation. As you are inhaling, feel the expansions of your belly, rib cage, and chest, and as you are exhaling, you feel the contractions of all three. Repeat this series several times. Release your breathing and feel the impact (Figure 1).

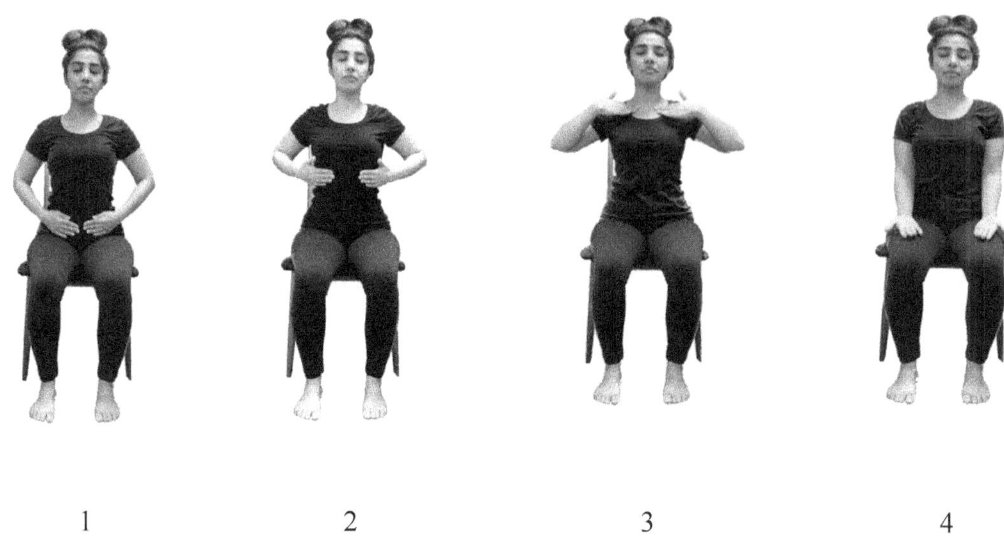

Figure 1: Dirgha Pranayama

🎧 **Warm-up: Sun breaths (Visit website to listen)**

-   On an inhale, swing your arms toward the sky, let your fingers and palms touch centered above your head, and on an exhale, bring your hands down into the prayer position in front of the center of your chest. Inhale, raise your arms up toward the sky and exhale, bring them down in front of your chest.

-   Repeat and coordinate your breath with your arm movements (Figure 2).

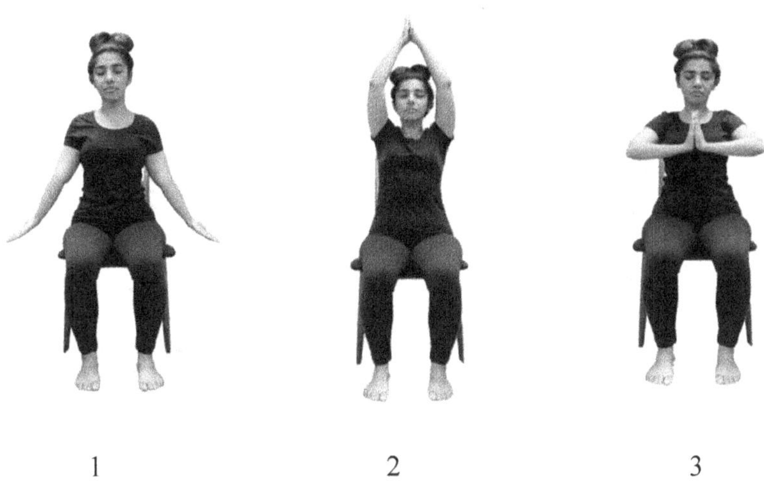

Figure 2: Sun Breaths

Posture steps for performing the Mountain Pose (Visit website to listen)

1- Stand straight with your feet parallel, rotate the sole of your right foot and place it next to the big toe of your left foot, then rotate your right foot back. This is hip-width apart. Inhale and exhale while lifting your toes up and down a few times to feel stability through the soles of your feet. Now balance your weight equally between the two feet. Straighten your knees but do not lock them. On an inhale, straighten your back. Exhale and bring your shoulders up, and then soften them back and down. Open your sternum. Feel the crown of your head reaching for the sky.

2- Inhale as you lift and extend your arms out to the sides and above your head into a V position. Relax your neck and keep your shoulders back and down. Hold this posture for a few seconds and feel grounded like a mountain.

3- To release, on an exhale, lower your arms down, relax and feel the effect of Tadasana (Figure 3).

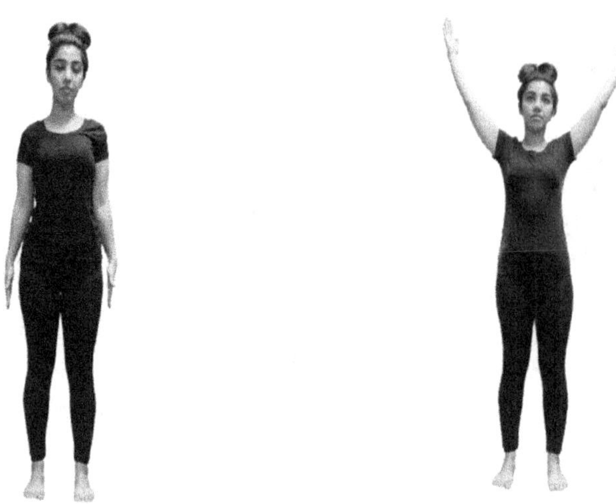

Figure 3: Mountain Pose (Tadasana)

Chapter 2

Section 1: Short Story: Moon

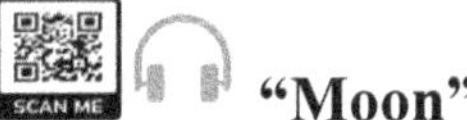 **"Moon"**

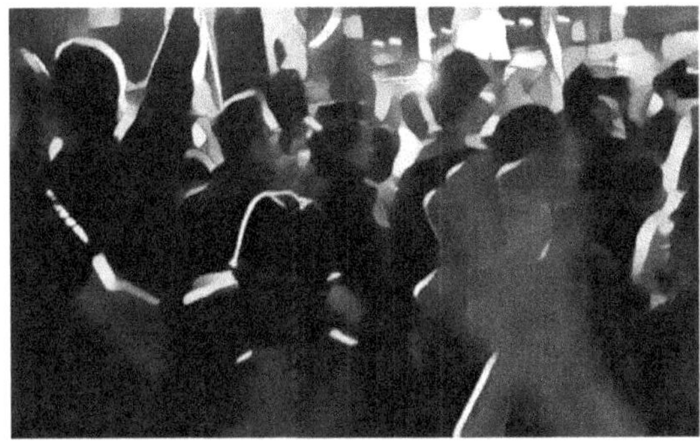 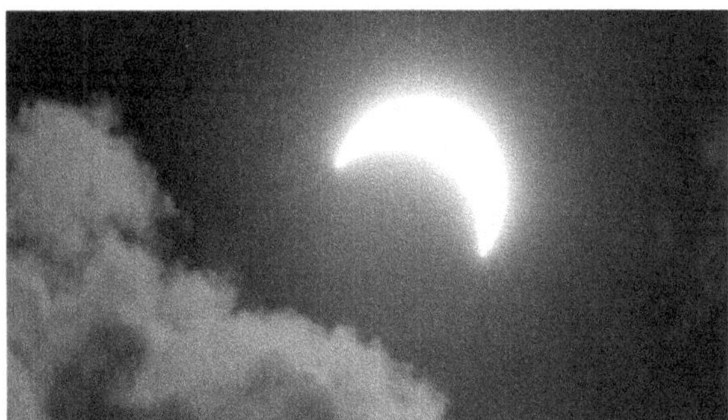

Once upon a time, Natalia was a bored l7 year old teenager. She asked her dad if she could have her first teenage party on the weekend. He agreed and she invited all her friends. Her friends came from far and near. It was the night of the party, and the half moon was in the sky. The music was playing, everybody was dancing, but Natalia was wondering who can come and dance with her to make a full moon. While she was wondering, a handsome nerdy boy approached her and said: "Would you like to dance?", she replied: "Maybe". Sam said: "Oh, come on, let's dance!". Natalia replied "Ok". They started to dance. While they were dancing, Sam said that "you shine like the moon in the sky. Natalia felt the full energy of his eyes and replied, "Thank you!". They held hands and kept dancing. After a while, Natalia stopped the music and clapped her hands and said: "Hey, girls! hey guys! welcome to my party, time to dance to "Jennifer& Pitbull", time to make a move, let's party." Everyone was so excited, and they started rocking to the "On the floor" song.

It is around 12 o'clock and the kids were still rocking and dancing away. Their cars lined the streets, and some were double-parked. Suddenly a policewoman knocked on the door. Her dad answered the door, the policewoman said: "I am sorry sir, but it is time to end the party. The cars outside are double parked and are a fire hazard because a fire engine will not be able to pass if there is a fire in the neighborhood". Natalia's dad replied "Ok" and then told the young people "The party will have to end". Quickly, all the young people got into their cars and went home. Natalia's dad breathed a sigh of relief as the last car left the neighborhood.

Section 2: Song and Lyrics: Moon

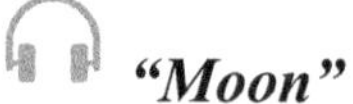 *"Moon"*

See the sky with a half moon

Hold my hand and we'll shine like a full moon

Put your hands in mine

You're my valentine

I've got a crush on you

You're so cute I'll tell you

Time to dance with Jennifer Pitbull

Stop, tonight don't be boring and dull

Let's shake it, dance till tomorrow

Let's forget about all sadness and sorrow

Put your hands in mine

Waste no time you're fine

I've got a crush on you

You're so cute I'll tell you

I love you the sky is the limit

Look at the moon, feel the spirit

Section 3: Museum of Reincarnation: Ludwig van Beethoven

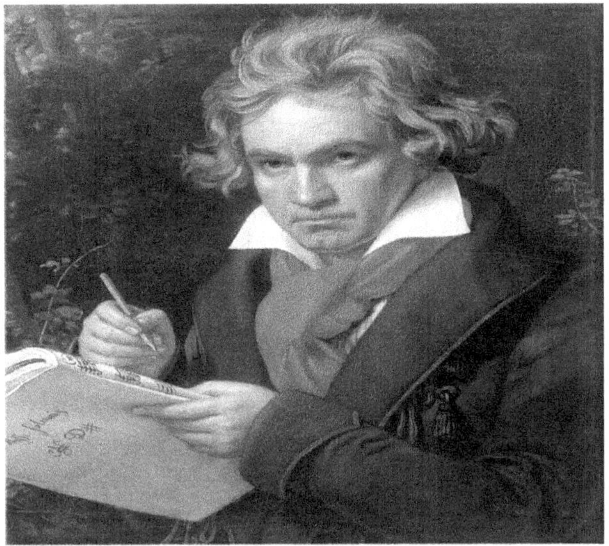

Wikipedia contributors, 2022, Ludwig van Beethoven

🎧 The biography part of the museum (Visit website to listen)

🎧 Visiting the museum (Visit website to watch and listen)

Museum Transcripts

a. Biography

Ludwig Van Beethoven (1770-1827) was born in Bonn, Germany, and is considered by many to be the greatest composer and pianist of the 18th and 19th centuries. His [23]genius was [24]apparent at an early age. By age 16, he traveled to Vienna to study with Mozart, the great composer, and pianist. At the height of his musical genius, Beethoven started to become [25]deaf. Despite his deafness and perhaps because of it, he continued to compose at a [26]furious rate. The Moonlight

---

[23] very great and rare natural ability or skill
[24] shown
[25] unable to hear
[26] extremely angry

Sonata was one of the most beautiful and [27]haunting of his compositions from this period of his

life ("Ludwig van Beethoven.," n.d.; Thayer & Krehbiel, (2020); Wikipedia contributors (2022)).

b. Paraphrased Quotations

A great poet, a great music, and singing with joy and passion are the keys to the world of art. A

fine poet is a gift of gold for the world. Music is the spirit of the creative life. "If you'll give

happiness and joy instead of sadness and sorrows to many others, then you're a happy fellow."

For the true artist, the sky is the limit. To sing a wrong note does not matter but waste no time

and do not sing without passion. When there is no passion, then the day-to-day routines of life is

boring and dull. So, listen to the notes of your heart and sing the melody of love with passion.

Share the melody of your heart with theirs (with the hearts of other people) and make a

symphony of love and peace in the world. My friend! never forget about the days we were

together and always be my friend. "Love demands all and has a right to all." (Ludwig van

Beethoven Quotes. (n.d.). BrainyQuote.com).

Section 4: Deepening our Cultural Understanding: "On the Floor, Singers"

"On the Floor, Singers"

"**Jennifer Lynn Lopez** (born July 24, 1969), also known by her nickname J.Lo, is an American

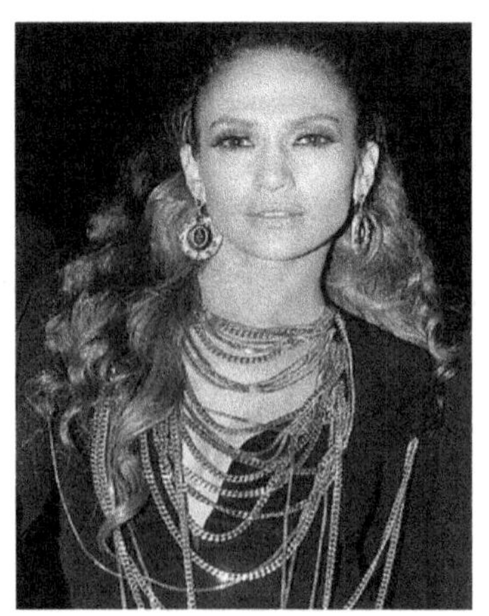

actress, singer, dancer, fashion designer, producer, and

businesswoman" with a Puerto Rican background. Her parents

were [28]relatively poor during her childhood, but with her

---

[27] beautiful, but in a sad way and often in a way that cannot be forgotten
[28] almost

[29]persistence and great [30]effort, she has become one of the most successful women in the world. While she was married to Alex Rodriguez, who also came from a [31]humble beginning and became one of the richest baseball players in the world, the [32]pair [33]stepped up with a [34]generous donation after being touched by an elementary school teacher's emotional post on Facebook about having to buy a student food which went [35]viral (France, 2019). The couple also helped to ensure that families got the food they needed amid the coronavirus pandemic.

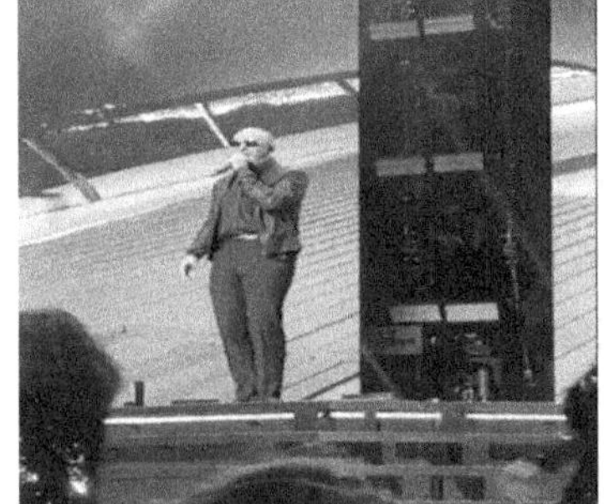

"**Armando Christian Pérez** (born January 15, 1981), known professionally as Pitbull, is an American rapper, singer, songwriter and record producer" ("Pitbull (rapper)," n.d.). He plays hard, and he works hard. When asked for his best investment tips, Pitbull said: "Don't be afraid to lose. Listen. And always [36]invest in yourself."

According to the biography "Pitbull: Mr. Worldwide," the rapper had a reason for wanting to be known after a particular [37]breed of dog."(Pitbulls) bite to lock," the book quotes him as saying. "The dog is too stupid to lose. And they're [38]outlawed in Dade County (Florida). They're basically everything that I am. It's been a [39]constant fight." **He is also [40]inspiring the next [41]generation to be successful like him.** Beyond recording music, Pitbull is using that

---

[29] someone who is persistent continues doing something
[30] physical or mental activity needed to achieve something
[31] poor or of a low social rank
[32] two people who have a romantic relationship or are doing something together
[33] to take action when there is a need or opportunity for it
[34] willing to give money, help, kindness, etc., especially more than is usual or expected
[35] used to describe something that quickly becomes very popular
[36] to put money, effort, time, etc. into something to make a profit or get an advantage
[37] a particular type of animal
[38] to make something illegal or unacceptable
[39] all the time
[40] to make someone feel that they want to do something and can do it
[41] all the people of about the same age within a society

passion for helping shape the future. He helped create the Sports Leadership and Management Academy, aka SLAM, a charter school in Miami with a sports-based curriculum (France, 2014). Miami rapper/songwriter Pitbull dropped a new single on Monday, turning the familiar sports chant "I Believe That We Will Win" into a pop anthem for the COVID-19 outbreak, with all proceeds from the song being donated to charity.

Section 5: Yoga Posture: Half-Moon

Ardha:half; Chandra: Moon; Asana

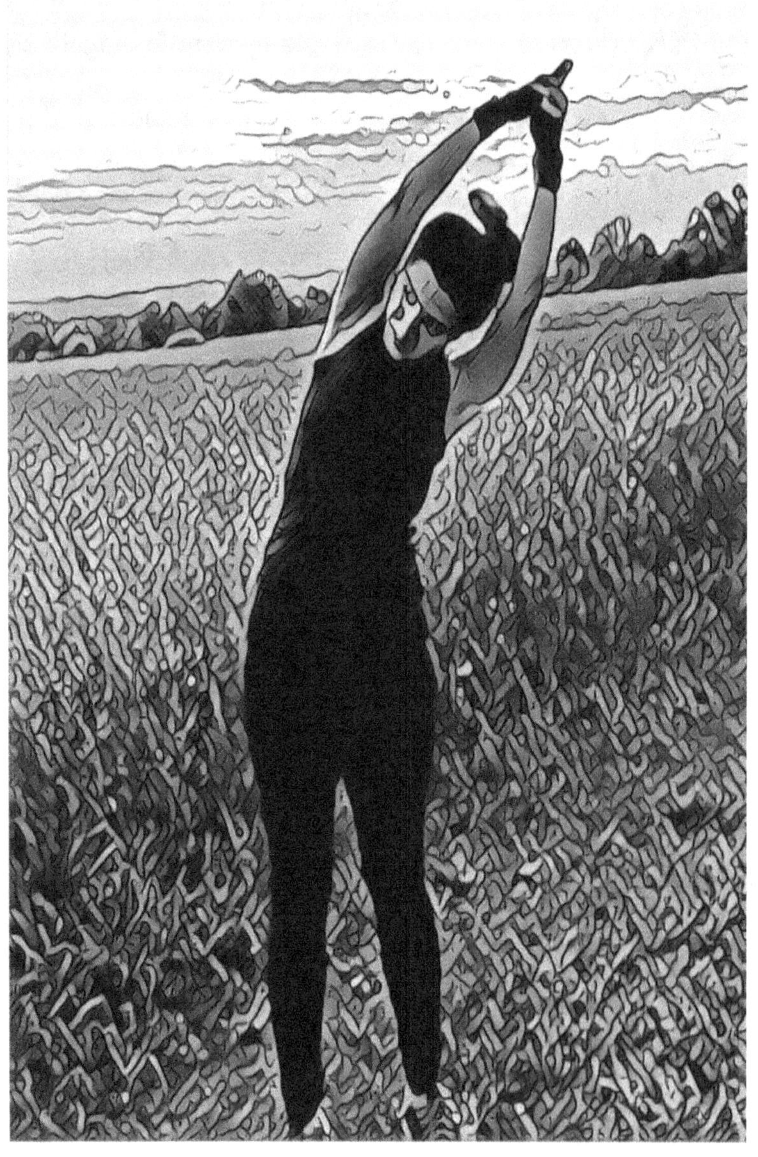

Follow your dreams, become who you are supposed to become, and shine like a moon in the sky!

Mythology of Ardha Chandrasana

This posture considers the energy of the moon as its great symbol. The significance of this asana is to channel the moon or lunar energy within the body. More than just the moon, the Chandra refers to something that is glittering and shining, a brilliant object that is illuminated by light on its own. In many traditional yogic texts and stories, the moon symbolizes one-half of the two polar energies in the body (Gaia, 2019).

The feminine energy of Chandra is only half of the energy in the universe. There is a second half of the energy, and it is the masculine energy. These two forces complete each other and are always searching for their compliment for completion. The idea of the complementary forces of the masculine and the feminine is found in cultures around the world, such as Mexico and Japan. In Teotihuacan, near Mexico City, there are huge pyramids known as the Pyramid of the Sun and the Pyramid of the Moon. The Moon is the counterpart that balances the sun. She represents cooling, calming, instinct, reflection, mystery, emotion, and the dream world. In Japan, Tsukuyomi-no-Mikoto is the moon god in Japanese mythology. The name "Tsukuyomi" is a compound of the Old Japanese words tsuku ("moon, month") and yomi ("reading, counting). An alternative interpretation is that his name is a combination of "moonlit night" and "looking, watching" (Kokugo Dai Jiten,1988).

Connection to the lesson

The girl of our story, Natalia, is a teenager with a lot of energy and trying to find the right chemistry with the others at her first teenage party. The restless energy of Chandra is familiar to all young people. There is a continuing search for balance for the powerful energies of the Chandra.

Cautionary notes

- Do not hold for a long period of time if you have any heart or circulatory issues

- Place your hands on your hips. If you have any injury to the affected area or if you have back problems

Yogic Breathing: Dirgha Pranayama
Meaning: Prana: air; life force; Yama: to restrain or hold back

Potential effects

Enhancement of complete and full breathing, decreasing stress and tension while calming the mind and the body, helping the lungs remain healthy by increasing the oxygen flow to the blood, it massages the abdominal organs, facilitating digestion, preparing you for a better learning experience.

Three Breathing Steps: (Visit website to listen)

1- Sit up straight with your shoulders back and down with relaxed abdominals.

2- Relax the face, close your mouth, and place your hands on your belly.

3- Breathe into your belly and feel it expands like a balloon. Repeat several times.

4- Now, put your hands to the sides of your rib cage and breathe into them, feeling the rib cage expand, and repeat several times.

5- Put your fingertips on your upper chest. Breathe into it and feel your hands lifting. Repeat several times.

6- Now, make a complete inhalation. As you are inhaling, feel the expansions of your belly, rib cage, and chest, and as you are exhaling, you feel the contractions of all three. Repeat this series several times (Refer to Figure 1 in Chapter 1).

Next, move into the warmup, which is the next section.

Warm-up: Arms overhead Stretch (Visit website to listen)

Stand with your feet wider than shoulder width. On an inhale, raise your hands over your head toward the sky and hold your hands as wide as your feet. Do not bend your elbows. On an exhale, stretch your arms behind your ears as is comfortable for you. Exhale to the right and inhale back to center. Exhale to the left and inhale back to center. Repeat moving from side to side in coordination with your breathing (Figure 1).

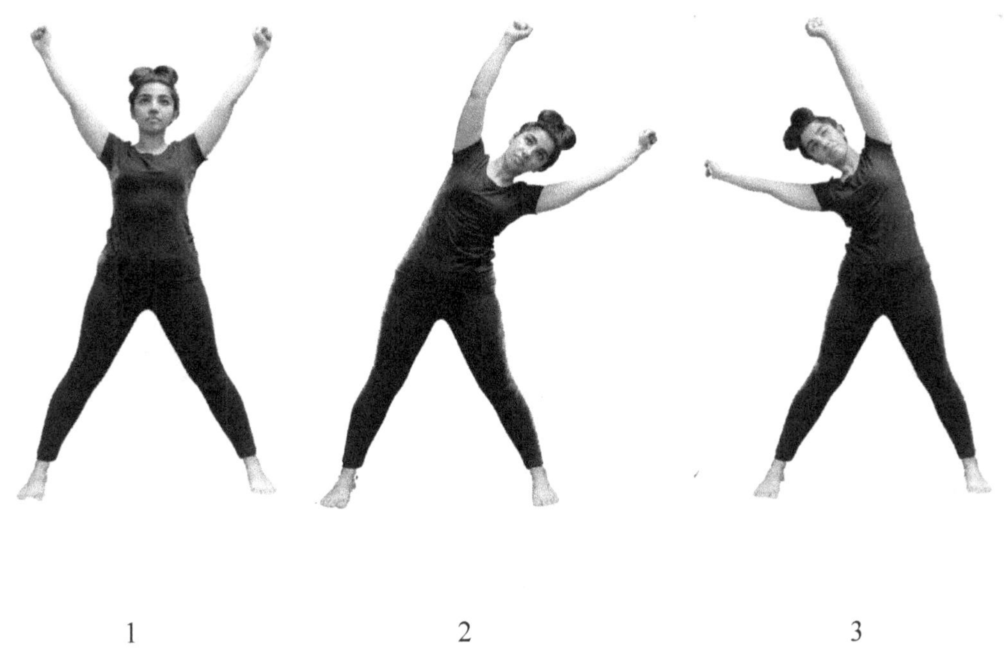

Figure 1: Arms Overhead Stretch

Posture steps for performing the half-moon pose (Visit website to listen)

1- While standing tall with your feet hip-width apart.

2- On an inhale, swing your arms over your head and clasp your fingers together with your index fingers pointing toward the sky. Ground the soles of your feet into the earth. Straighten your back. Drop the tailbone. Roll your shoulders back and down. Stand tall.

3- Inhale and switch the weight toward your left foot and lengthen toward your right side. Distribute your weight on both feet. Keep your shoulders and hips squared to the front.

4- To release, exhale, relax your arms down by your sides, feel the difference, and feel the effect of Ardha Chandrasana (half-moon pose). Take a few breaths and perform on the other side (Figure 2).

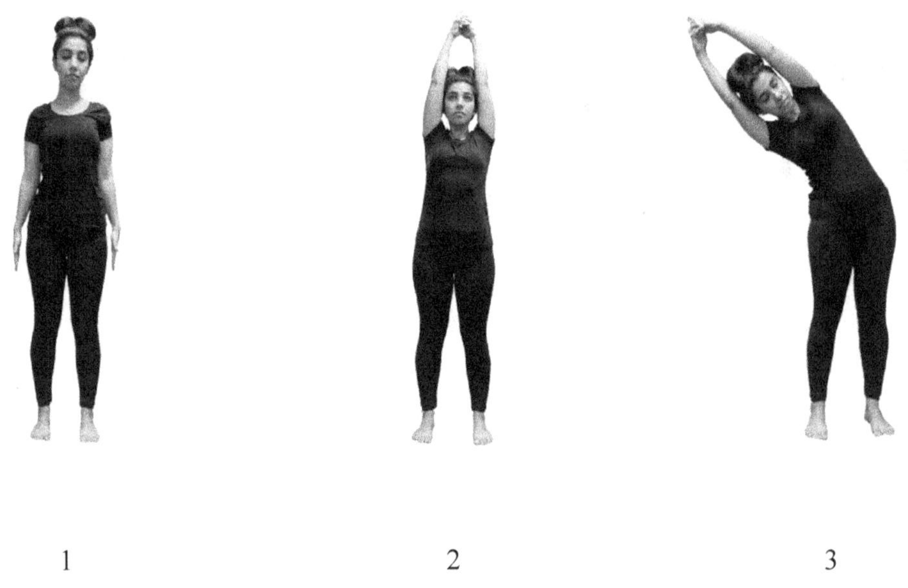

Figure 2: Half-Moon (Ardha Chandrasana)

Chapter 3

Section 1: Short Story: We are Superstars

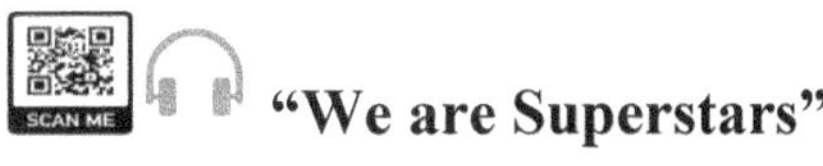 **"We are Superstars"**

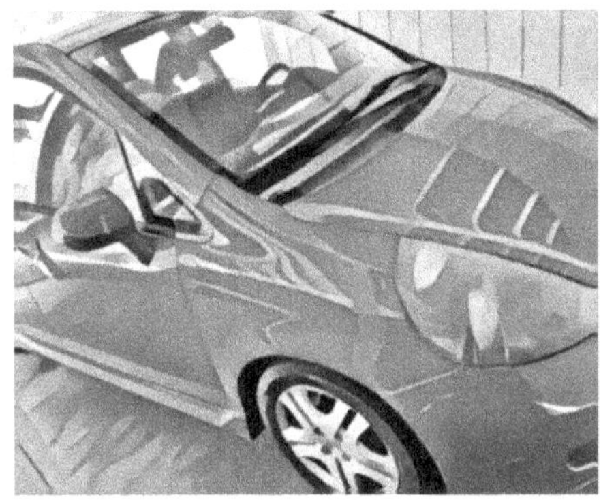 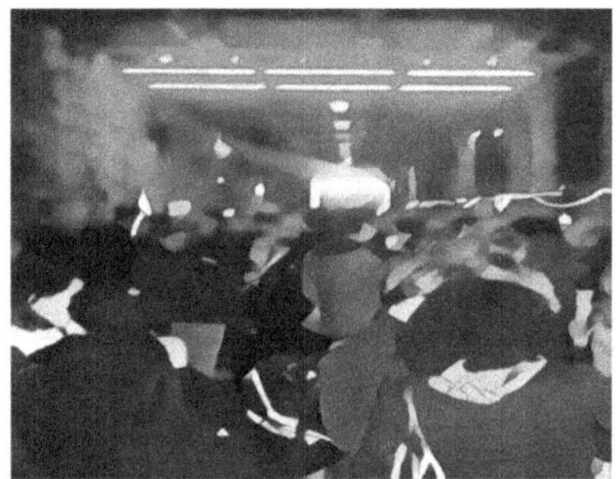

Natalia is now 18 years old; She has recently received her driver's license. She is working afterschool and has bought her first car with the help of her dad. She is so excited about her new little red car.

One Saturday night, Natalia and her friend Sara decided to go to a party. They dressed up and the two beautiful young girls got into the Natalia's small red car and headed toward the party. They imagined their little red car was a luxurious car. They listened to the music in the car, sang and danced on their way to the party. They named their little red car "Luxy". They were feeling like Cinderellas going to the Ball. They arrived at the party. They had a drink and sipped it all night. After a while they started talking about their luxury car and they decided to pretend that they were superstars the whole night. Suddenly, they noticed the prince, a young man with a smile and an attractive style. Sara said excitedly to Natalia "The prince is smiling at you; he has a crush on you." Natalia told Sara: "Let us not doubt ourselves, we are eagles, we are superstars, he can wait." Then they burst into laughter and started dancing. The young man approached Natalia and asked her "Shall we dance?", Natalia replied "No, thank you. It is close to midnight, and we must go home." The young man was so polite and told Natalia "No problem, please enjoy your night". Then Natalia and Sara got into Luxy and went home. When they got home, they were exhausted, and soon fell asleep. In the morning they woke up and remembered the story of last night. Sara told Natalia "I think we got too carried away with our Superstar story, girl, it's sad, you missed your chance to get his number." Natalia said to Sara "I did, he was both polite and handsome, but don't worry, we are superstars. We can always have fun without him in our Luxy, we are eagles and we do not doubt our inner regal. You are a superstar. Don't wonder who you are!" While they were laughing and singing "We are Superstars" they got out of their bed to have breakfast.

Section 2: Song and Lyrics: We Are Superstars

"We Are Superstars"

Last night Sara and I went to a party

with my little red car

We danced, and we thought

that we were superstars

At the party we noticed someone's smile

who had been watching us for a while

This guy is cute and awesome

He is smiling at you

He is cool and handsome

Aren't we 2 superstars?

"So, he is not worthy of us at all,

time to leave in our luxury car?"

We both burst into a long laughter

Dancing and went home soon after

In the morning waking

from a deep long slumber

Regretting not having this guy's number

But who cares?

We are still superstars

We can have fun without him

in our luxury car

"We dream big, fly high like an eagle, we don't doubt our beauty and inner regal"

Section 3: Museum of Reincarnation: Marie Curie

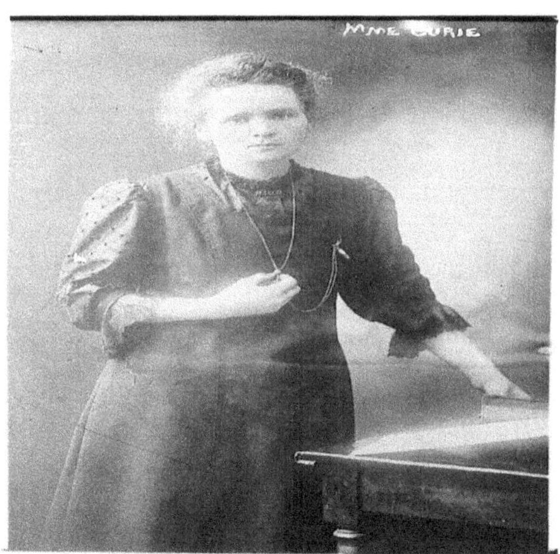

Bain News Services. *Marie Curie*

🎧 The biography part of the museum (Visit website to listen)

🎧 Visiting the museum (Visit website to watch and listen)

Museum Transcripts

a. Biography

Marie Skłodowska Curie (1867–1934) was a Polish and naturalized-French physicist and chemist who [42]conducted [43]pioneering research on [44]radioactivity. The [45]discovery of radioactivity by Henri Becquerel in 1896 [46]inspired Marie and her husband in their [47]brilliant research and analyses, which led to the [48]isolation of polonium, named after the country of Marie's birth, and radium. She won her first Nobel Prize in physics in [49]collaboration with her husband for the study of [50]spontaneous radiation, and she won her second Nobel prize in Chemistry for her research in radioactivity ("Marie Curie.," n.d.; Charles River Editors (2018); Wikipedia contributors (2022).

b. Paraphrased Quotations

Who cares about the personal life of people? What matters are ideas. To be a superstar, each of us must work for our own improvement. We must have perseverance and, above all, confidence in ourselves. We must believe that we are worthy and gifted for something and that this thing must be attained. When you are working with passion, you smile, and you burst into laughter because it makes you rejoice like a child. Have passion and enjoy the present moment by focusing on your passion, or you will regret losing grace. I am one of those who thought, like Nobel, that humanity will draw more good than evil from new discoveries. One never notices

---

[42] did, performed
[43] being the first to do or use a new idea
[44] the quality that some atoms have of producing a type of energy that can be very harmful to health
[45] Finding for the first time
[46] to make someone feel that they want to do something and can do it
[47] Great, extremely intelligent
[48] Separation
[49] the situation of two or more people working together
[50] happening or done in a natural, often sudden way, without any planning or without being forced

what has been done; one can only see what remains to be done. Have no fear at all of perfection; you will never reach it. (Marie Curie Quotes. (n.d.). BrainyQuote.com).

Section 4: Deepening our Cultural Understanding: Oprah, Beyoncé, Jolie

Oprah

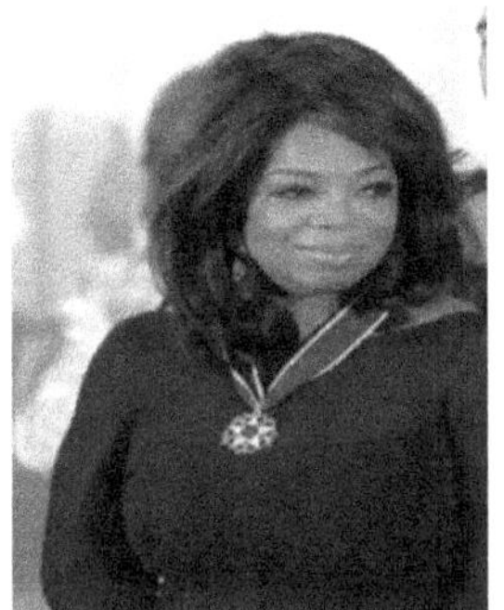

Oprah, 66, is only the third woman in history to own her own television and film production studio, joining Mary Pickford and Lucille Ball. She proved that the wildest dreams could come true with hard work and determination, [51]faith, and persistence. She's journeyed from being a poor child to an international icon whose influence goes beyond the world of television into social [52]awareness, publishing, film, philanthropy[53] , and education. (Mayor, 2000), Oprah was an honors student in high school, earned a full scholarship for college, and is now a billionaire that millions look up to and admire." (Hall, 2014), Oprah Winfrey donated $10 million to coronavirus relief.

Beyoncé

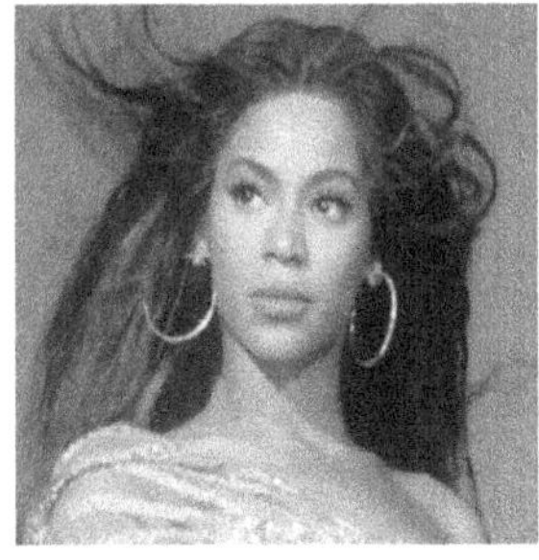

"The singer, in a rare 2016 interview with Elle, explained her decision to define the word "feminist" within the lyrics of her single "Flawless." "I put the definition of feminist in my song and on my tour, not for [54]propaganda but to give [55]clarity to the true meaning. I'm not really sure

---

[51] belief
[52] information
[53] the activity of helping the poor, especially by giving them money
[54] information, ideas often only giving one part of an argument, that are published, with the intention of influencing people's opinions
[55] the quality of being clear and easy to understand

people know or understand what a feminist is, but it's very simple. It's someone who believes in [56]equal [57]rights for men and women," she told Elle." (Jang, 2017). She also has donated $6m for mental health and other initiatives during the Covid-19 pandemic.

Angelina Jolie

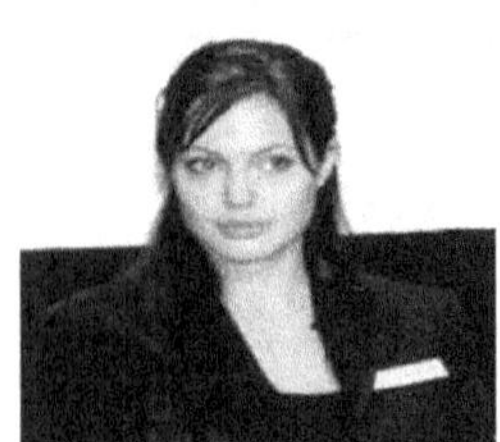

Angelina, "Hollywood's most famous actresses and [58]philanthropist" (Trejo, 2019). "She gave a speech at the 2015 African Union Summit where she spoke about the importance of women's rights nationwide." (Jang, 2017). She also donated $1M to help feed hungry children during the pandemic.

"There is a [59]global [60]epidemic of [61]violence against women — both within conflict zones and within societies at peace, and it is still treated as a lesser crime and lower [62]priority," Jolie said. "We need [63]policies for long-term [64]security that are [65]designed by women, focused on women, [66]executed by women — not at the expense of men, or instead of men, but alongside and with men. "She continued, "There is no greater pillar of [67]stability than a strong, free, and [68]educated woman. And there is no more inspiring role model than a man who respects and [69]cherishes women and [70]champions their [71]leadership" (Jang, 2017).

---

[56] the same in amount, number, or size
[57] the legal authority to publish, copy, or make available a work such as a book, movie, recording, or work of art
[58] a person who helps the poor, especially by giving them money
[59] worldwide
[60] Widespread; a particular problem that seriously affects many people at the same time
[61] actions or words that are intended to hurt people
[62] something that you do or deal with first because it is more important or urgent than other things
[63] diplomacy
[64] safety
[65] selected
[66] Do, perform
[67] a situation in which something is not likely to move or change
[68] having learned a lot at school or college and having a good level of knowledge
[69] To love and protect, to care
[70] To support
[71] Control and management

Section 5: Yoga Posture: Eagle

Yoga Posture: Eagle (Asana: Garudasana)
Gardua: Eagle; Asana: posture

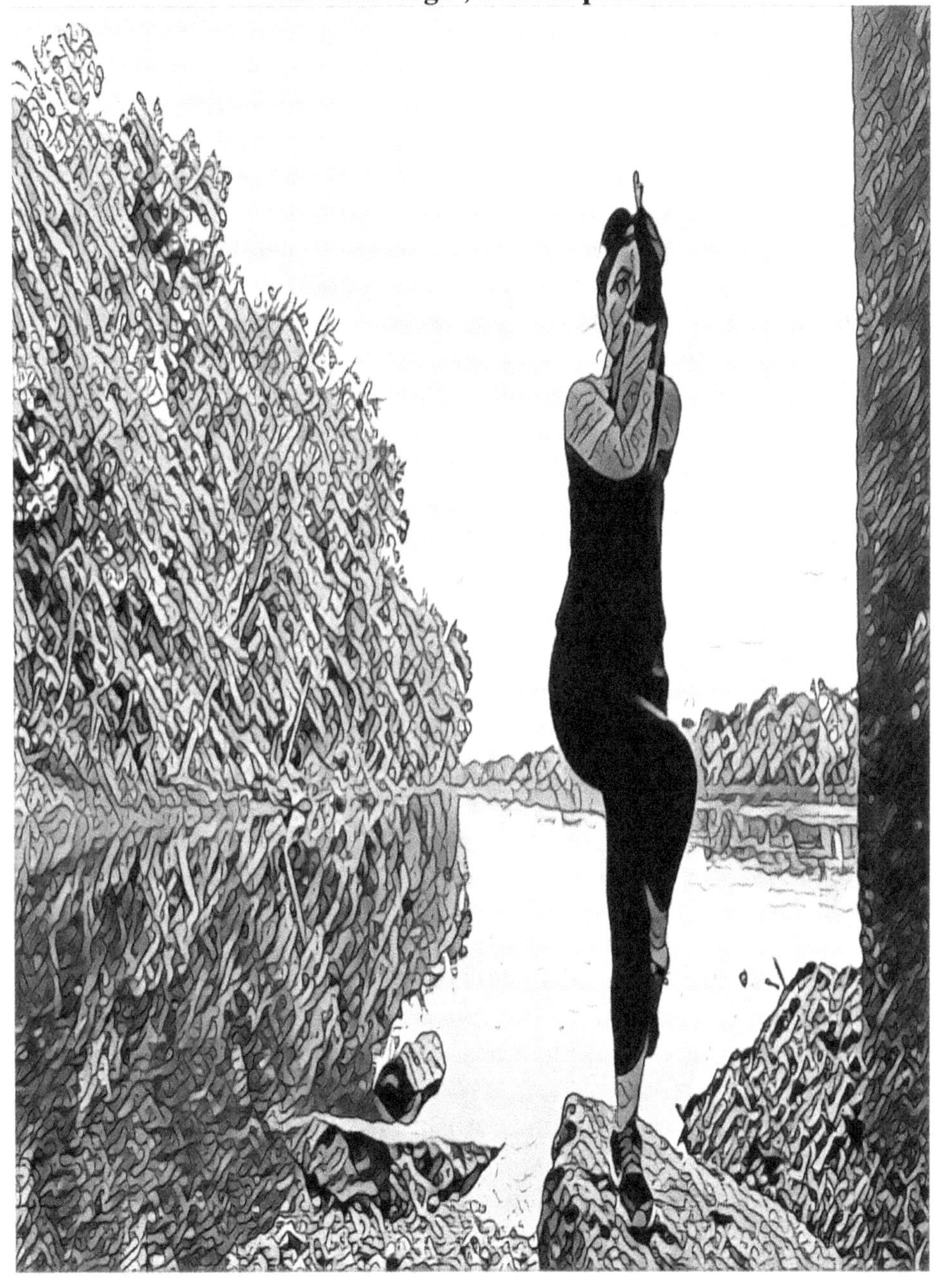

Open the sharp vision of your heart, dream big, fly high, and do not be afraid to become what you are supposed to be, be an eagle!

Mythology of Garudasana

The Eagle is the king of birds, a symbol of power and victory. It is an emblem of victory in battle and the triumph of spirit over matter. Today the person of outstanding intelligence, who has lofty thoughts and conceives of high-flying projects, is often compared to an eagle. The eagle depicts the age-old conflict between power of the mind (soaring eagle) and matter (temptation). Ask yourself: "Can I see my struggle clearly (sharp vision)? What is my target? (Can I act at the right time and at the right place)" (Radha, 2006).

According to Paul Tillich (2008), it requires courage to be an eagle. The Eagle is a strong and regal bird and known in various myths as one of God's messengers. As you sit deeply into the eagle pose, you can imagine yourself flying between the earthly and spiritual planes, with an Eagle Eye that takes in the greater perspective of life. *Garudasana* (Eagle pose) demands great focus and patience, as does living a life in accordance with Spirit. It is easy to get bogged down with the challenges of life (or of this pose!), but a calm connection with the Divine can help you soar on to your journey.

Many cultures have associated the eagle with the most important of their gods. In Egypt, the solar symbolism was shared by the falcon and the eagle, and this heavenly principle is the divine vision. The symbol of the United States is the eagle. Many cultures have adopted the symbol of the eagle, and even in modern times, Austria has the double-headed eagle as its special emblem. The arms of Mexico show the eagle with the serpent. Aristotle tells a story of the eagle's fabulous eyesight, which allowed it to look directly at the sun. This story was later expanded to symbolize Christ as the eagle who could look directly at his father (Hatha yoga).

Connection to the lesson

In this song, the girl of the story, Natalia, is switching between different feelings and planes of imagination. Starting a relationship with the boy (temptation) and feeling the power of independence (soaring eagle).

Cautionary notes

If you have a persistent heart issue, high/low blood pressure, or weak knees, please consult your physicians and avoid holding the posture for a long period of time.

Yogic Breathing: Dirgha Pranayama (Visit website to listen)
Meaning: Prana: air; life force; Yama: to restrain or hold back

Potential effects

Enhancement of complete and full breathing, decreasing stress and tension while calming the mind and the body, helping the lungs remain healthy by increasing the oxygen flow to the blood, it massages the abdominal organs, facilitating digestion, preparing you for a better learning experience

Three Breathing Steps:

1- Sit up straight with your shoulders back and down with relaxed abdominals.

2- Relax the face, close your mouth, and place your hands on your belly.

3- Breathe into your belly and feel it expands like a balloon. Repeat several times.

4- Now, put your hands to the sides of your rib cage and breathe into them, feeling the rib cage expand and repeat several times.

5- Put your fingertips on your upper chest. Breathe into it and feel your hands lifting. Repeat several times.

6- Now, make a complete inhalation. As you are inhaling, feel the expansions of your belly, rib cage, and chest, and as you are exhaling, you feel the contractions of all three. Repeat this series several times (Refer to Figure 1 in Chapter 1).

Next, move into the warmup, which is the next section.

🎧 Warm-up: Balancing knee (Visit website to listen)

1- Stand tall in Tadasana and keep your feet parallel and close to each other. Shift your weight from your left foot to right and from your right foot to your left several times.

 2- On an inhale, sweep your arms to the sides, palms facing down.

 3- On an exhale, raise your left knee up in front of you until your thigh is at a 90-degree angle with the floor. On an inhale, bring your foot down. Feel the difference and repeat on the other side (Figure 1).

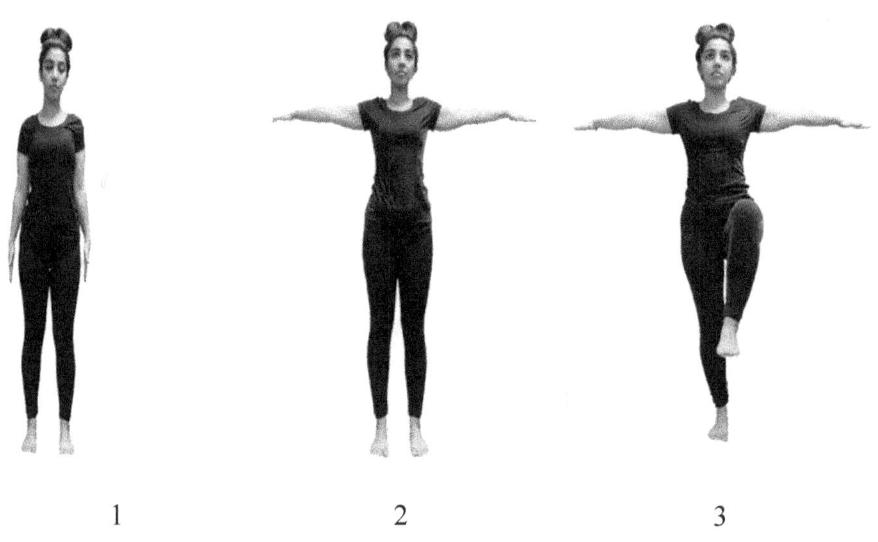

1   2   3

Figure 1: Balancing Knee

Posture steps of Garudasana (Eagle Pose): (Visit website to listen)

1- Stand tall with your feet hip-width apart and parallel to each other.

2- On an exhale, blend both knees, until you feel the engagement of your quad muscles.

3- Inhale and shift your weight onto your right foot and lift your left foot. On an exhale, rotate your left knee out and high and swing it over your right leg. While maintaining the balance, on an inhale, bend your left knee as comfortable. Keep your pelvis neutral, and your hips squared and parallel.

4- On an inhale, swipe your arms to the sides and then cross your right arm over your left. On an exhale, bend your elbows and lift your hands in front of your face.

5- Inhale while slowly bending your right knee and let your hips sink down a bit while pressing your legs and arms together. Keep breathing and balance your torso until your elbows are just above your knees. Hold the posture for a few seconds.

6- To release, exhale, uncross your arms and then your legs. Relax, rest, feel the effect of Garudasana (the eagle pose) and repeat on the other side (Figure 2).

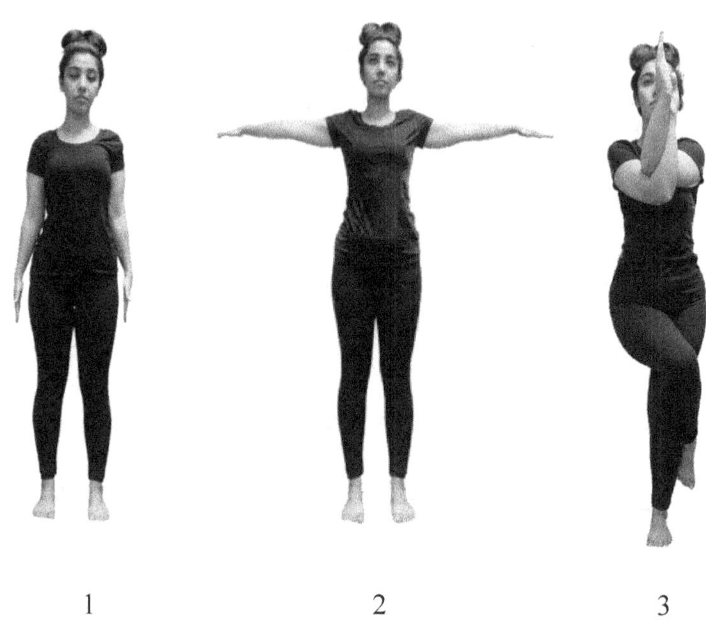

Figure 2: Eagle (Garudasana)

Chapter 4

Section 1: Short Story: 411

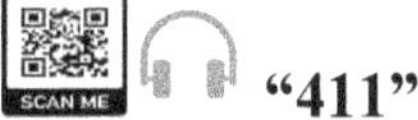 "411"

Natalia and her family have recently moved from California to Boston, Massachusetts where she is going to college.

One day while walking her dog, [72]Assal, in [73]Peter's Park near her home, she remembers her friend Sara. She misses her a lot, and she remembers them being 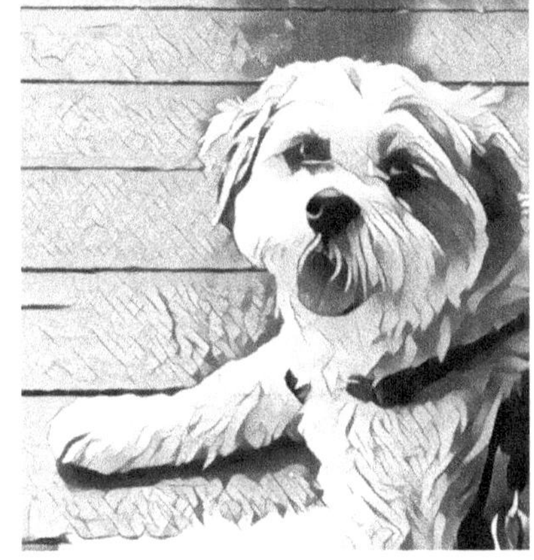 superstars in her little red car. A smile appears on her face as she remembers the fun times with Sara. She feels so proud of herself for being a top student at Boston College. She feels great pride because she overcame all the challenges to become an educated woman and to make her dad and family proud.

While in the park she stops at a stand where a charity [74]organization is selling hand-made necklaces to help children with special needs. She buys a necklace with her name on it. A young man whose name is Garcia is standing behind her and overhears her conversation. Garcia orders a necklace for himself to impress Natalia. As she is leaving, she is listening to a song on her headphones and humming the lyrics "I sit in the glorious chair of life, I am not afraid of challenges and strife!" and she is imagining the "chair pose" of yoga while she is singing along with the lyrics. Suddenly Assal begins to bark. Then, Garcia approached Natalia and asked her, "Hola, Señorita, May I talk to you?" Natalia replied, "Yes". Garcia asked curiously, "how are

---

[72] Means honey in Persian (Farsi)
[73] Peter's Park is a popular dog park in Boston, MA
[74] a group of people who work together in an organized way for

you? What's new with you today? Are you new to the neighborhood? Where are you from?".

Natalia replied, "Yes". Garcia asked curiously, "how are you? What's new with you today? Are

you new to the neighborhood? Where are you from?". Natalia replied, "I am from California".

Garcia said enthusiastically, "I have heard that California is beautiful, and I have seen pictures of

the Golden Gate Bridge. I have also heard that all Cali girls are smart. and beautiful just like

you." Natalia replied suspiciously, "You are such a sweet talker." Garcia said passionately,

"Natalia, I am not trying to fool you; I am saying this from the bottom of my heart.". Then he

asked, "May I call you? What is your 411?" Natalia replied, "Here is my number, but I must

warn you; My zodiac sign is Scorpio and Scorpio women are serious and independent, their mind

is tough, and their heart is so tender". Garcia said, "I admire your character my lady,". Then he

asked, "Could we meet for a cup of Chai? If you agree we can meet this Saturday at 6:00 pm at

Copley square?" Natalia replied, "Ok, Now, I must leave. See you later." Garcia replied

passionately "bye, please take care."

Later, they start dating and she falls in love with Garcia. One year passes and one day

Garcia explains that he must go on a short business trip to China. He tells Natalia that he needs to

borrow some money from her to make this business deal in China. He said, "Natalia, I will make

a lot of money and when I return, we can be married."

Natalia replied, "OH, Garcia, don't worry, we are going to make a life together and I want to

help you. No problem. I will give you the money from my savings."

Garcia said, "Thank you, sweetie. When I get back, I will have a surprise for you."

Natalia gives him all her savings. A few days later, Garcia leaves from Logan international

Airport for his trip to Wuhan, China.

Section 2: Song and Lyrics: 411

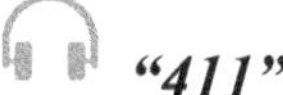 *"411"*

I sit in the glorious chair of life

I am not afraid of challenges and strife

Hola, señorita

Hey, missy what's new?

I am fine, how about you?

I am better now because I am seeing you

Oh, it's so kind of you

Do you have any idea, I am falling in love with ye

You've got no idea I have fallen in love with ye

Tell me where you're from señorita Natalia?

I am from California señor Garcia

Oh, I've heard the Golden Gate in Cali is so wonderful

I also heard Cali girls are beautiful

Oh, Sir, that's kind of you, You're a sweet talker too

Ok, Now, give me your 411

who knows maybe you're the one

Wait, just a minute, senior

here is my phone number,

My sign is Scorpio and

I was born in November

Never forget my mind is tough

my heart is tender

Missy I strongly recommend that

we surely meet up this weekend

Ok, tell me what time and where?

At 6, at Copley Art Square

Ok, Bye-bye See you later

Adios, Hasta Luego sweetie,

please please be well and take care

Section 3: Museum of Reincarnation: George Washington

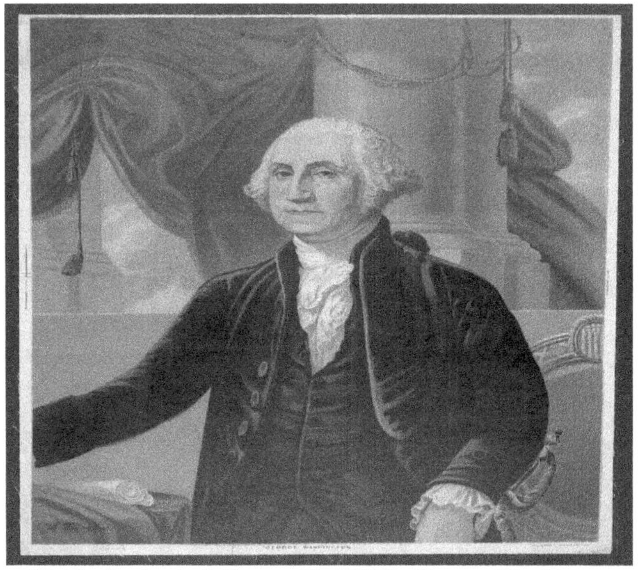

Weidenbach, A. & Stuart, G. (1876), George Washington

The biography part of the museum (Visit website to listen)

Visiting the museum (Visit website to watch and listen)

Museum Transcripts

a. Biography

George Washington (1732- 1799) was a [75]military leader, [76]statesman, and the founding father of the United States. Washington was [77]elected as the first president of the U.S and served two terms from 1789 to 1797. He was first elected to the House of Burgess (representative) of the state of Virginia and was selected as a [78]delegate to the [79]constitutional [80]convention. He was the head of the constitutional convention of 1787, which established the U.S. Constitution and a [81]federal government. He was selected by the convention to lead the continental army in the war for independence from Great Britain. He led the army to [82]victory, and the Peace Treaty of Paris was signed in 1783 ("George Washington.," n.d.).

b. Paraphrased Quotations

Let's start with two facts about me. Do you have an idea that I fell in love with agriculture and became an expert in it? My love for the land began with my careful planting and harvesting of the crops. I experimented with different crops and found those that were the most useful. I discovered that if you give love to the land, the land will give you love in return. My second passion was for peace among nations, and who knows what the fruits of peace and history will be? I met a French general, and we made peace. 100 years later, the French government gifted the United States the Statue of Liberty to support peace and immigration.

---

[75] fighting forces
[76] a politician or government official who is respected and experienced
[77] chose
[78] a person chosen or elected by a group to speak, vote, etc. for them, especially at a meeting
[79] relating to or following the rules of the US Constitution
[80] a large formal meeting of people who do a particular job or have a similar interest
[81] relating to the central government
[82] winning

When you are a peace seeker, a passionate one, and you have spirit, you can do anything. When perseverance and spirit meet up with knowledge, wonders happen in all ages. Knowledge is surely, in every country, the basis of public happiness. But do not forget through your journey, you need to make mistakes to learn and to be successful. I strongly recommend not looking back at your mistakes unless you can learn a useful lesson. My last advice is "Observe good faith and justice towards all nations, cultivate peace and harmony with all." (120 George Washington Quotes to Celebrate His Place In History, Hannah Hutyra, 2019)

Section 4: Deepening our Cultural Understanding: Harassment

"Harassment"

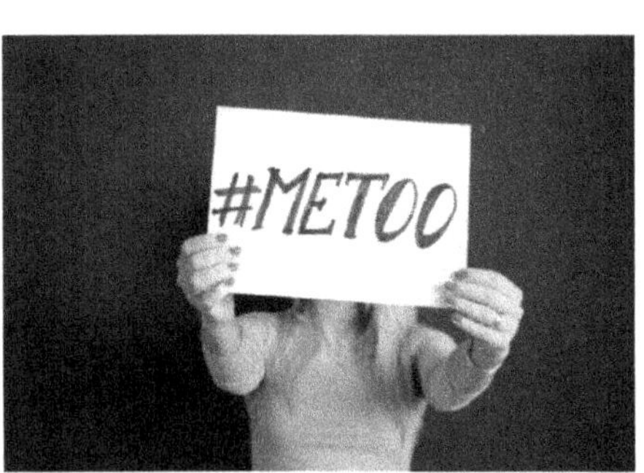

Street harassment is mainly sexual harassment that [83]consists of unwanted comments, [84]gestures, [85]honking, [86]wolf-whistling, [87]catcalling, exposure, stalking, persistent sexual advances, and touching by strangers in public areas such as streets, shopping malls, and public transportation.

[88]According to an article by the non-profit organization Stop Street, harassment can also include [89]persistent [90]requests for someone's name, number, destination, or other personal information (411) after the victim has already denied the requests. The practice of street harassment is rooted in power and control and is often a reflection of societal discrimination.

---

[83] a movement of the hands, arms, or head, etc. to express an idea or feeling
[84] Made up
[85] it makes a short, loud sound
[86] a whistle (= sound made by blowing air through the lips) sometimes made by a man when he sees a woman, he finds sexually attractive
[87] make a whistle, shout, or comment of a sexual nature to a woman passing by
[88] Based on
[89] continuous
[90] Asking for

In 2014, researchers from Cornell University and Hollaback conducted the largest international cross-cultural study of street harassment. The data suggests that the majority of females have their first street harassment experience during [91]puberty. (Whittaker & Kowalski, 2015).

Fortunately, many common street harassment behaviors are already illegal in the USA. In fact, since at least the late 1880s, some women have used these laws to report street harassers to the police.

Section 5: Yoga Posture: Chair

Yoga Posture: Standing Squat/Chair Pose (Asana: Utkatasana)
Utakata: Powerful, exceeding the usual measure; asana: posture

Dream big, sit proud and strong on the glorious chair of your dream!

---

[91] the period during which adolescents reach sexual maturity and become capable of reproduction

Mythology of Utkatasana

Sit inside the glorious purpose of your life and find strength with the chair pose. The name comes from the Sanskrit words *utkaṭa*, meaning "gigantic, powerful and proud" (Sjoman, 1999).ß

This pose follows the struggles of Rama, a divine prince, following his exile from the kingdom by his father. With courage and strength, he overcomes many struggles and challenges, and after fourteen years in exile, Rama returns to his birthplace to be crowned king and assume his rightful place on the throne. Of course, this myth is concerned with the theme of *utkata:* power, courage, and ferocity, all embodied in Rama. A throne is a type of chair reserved for the powerful that brings feelings of pride and the power of positive affirmations and gratitude (Kanzar, 2018). The significance of a throne chair is such that many of these thrones - such as China's Dragon Throne - survive today as historical examples of the nation's history.

Connection to the lesson

In this lesson, Natalia is proud and powerful when she is talking to Garcia. She is entering a college in Boston, and she feels so proud about it. She is so happy because she has overcome all academic challenges. And she feels she is entering a new period in her social life. (She is becoming familiar with Garcia and the positive affirmation that she is a Scorpio and independent).

Cautionary notes

Do not hold the posture for a long period of time If you have low, high blood pressure, heart issues, or weak knees.

Yogic Breathing: Dirgha Pranayama

Meaning: Prana: air; life force; Yama: to restrain or hold back

Potential effects

Enhancement of complete and full breathing, decreasing stress and tension while calming the mind and the body, helping the lungs remain healthy by increasing the oxygen flow to the blood, it massages the abdominal organs, facilitating digestion, preparing you for a better learning experience.

Three Breathing Steps: (Visit website to listen)

1- Sit up straight with your shoulders back and down with relaxed abdominals.

2- Relax the face, close your mouth, and place your hands on your belly.

3- Breathe into your belly and feel it expands like a balloon. Repeat several times.

4- Now, put your hands to the sides of your rib cage and breathe into them, feeling the rib cage expand, and repeat several times.

5- Put your fingertips on your upper chest. Breathe into it and feel your hands lifting. Repeat several times.

6- Now, make a complete inhalation. As you are inhaling, feel the expansions of your belly, rib cage, and chest, and as you are exhaling, you feel the contractions of all three. Repeat this series several times (Refer to Figure 1 in Chapter 1).

Warm-up: Torso Cat and Dog (Visit website to listen)

1- While sitting on your chair and placing the palms of your hands on your laps, on an inhale, expand your chest and arch your back. Ground your butt into the chair and feel the stretch. On an exhale, round your back while bending forward and drop your chin and feel the stretch. Inhale, expand your chest and arch your back. Exhale, round your back, bend forward and drop the chin.

2- Repeat the Torso cat and dog several times while coordinating your breath (Figure 1).

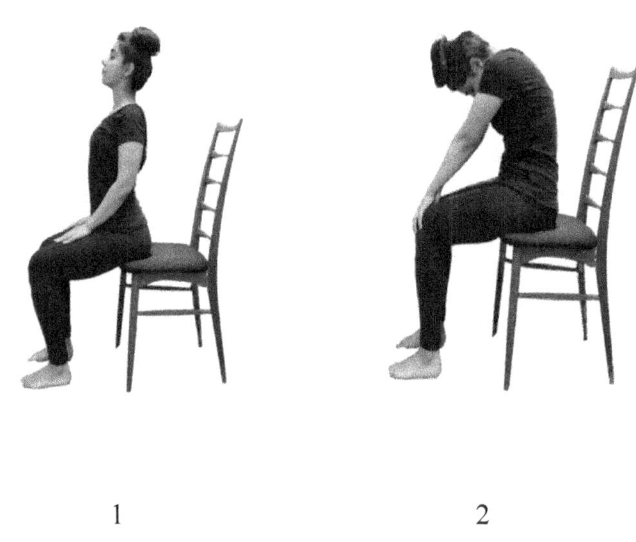

1   2

Figure 1: Torso Cat and Dog

Posture steps for Chair pose/ Standing Squat (Utkatasana), (Visit website to listen)

1- Stand tall in the Mountain pose with your feet hip-width apart.

2- On an inhale, slowly bend your knees and lower your hips. Gradually bow your back while maintaining the length in your waist. Allow your hips to sink to engage your front thighs and feel the stretch in your hamstrings, if you feel any discomfort raise your hips and take the pressure off your knees. Do not let the knees extend over your toes. Maintain the arch in your back.

3- On an inhale, sweep your arms in front of you parallel to the floor, palms facing down. Roll your shoulders back and down. Keep breathing and hold the pose for a few seconds.

4- To release, ground yourself firmly through your feet and come up and then allow your arms to sink down by your sides. Relax and feel the effect of Utkatasana, the chair pose (Figure 2).

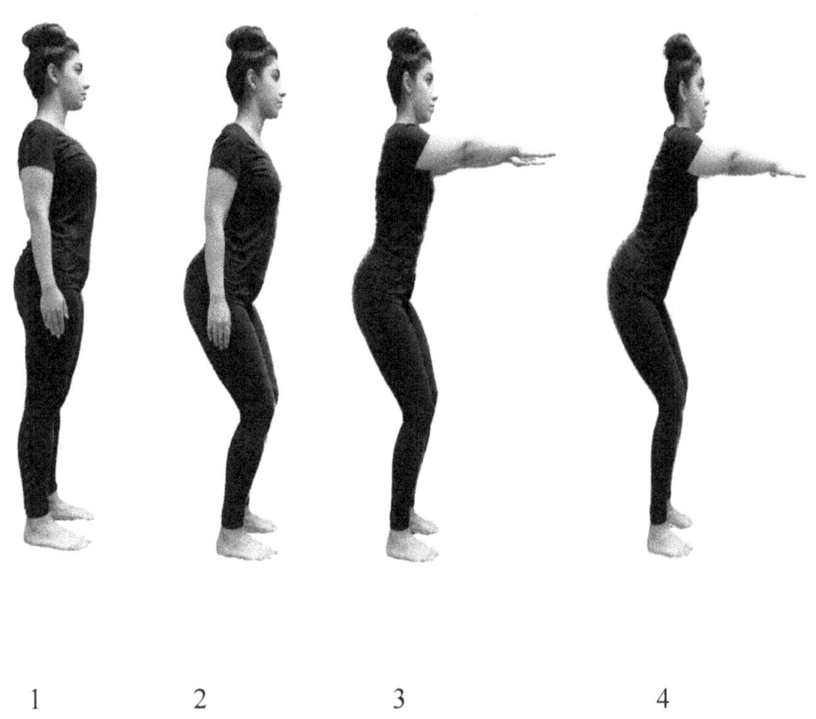

Figure 2: Chair Pose/Standing Squat (Utkatasana)

Chapter 5

Section 1: Short Story: Waiting and Waiting for You

 **"Waiting and Waiting for You"**

It is December 2019; it is almost time for Garcia to return home. One night, Natalia

receives a call from Garcia. He tells her, "I am ill, and I am in the hospital, I will return as soon

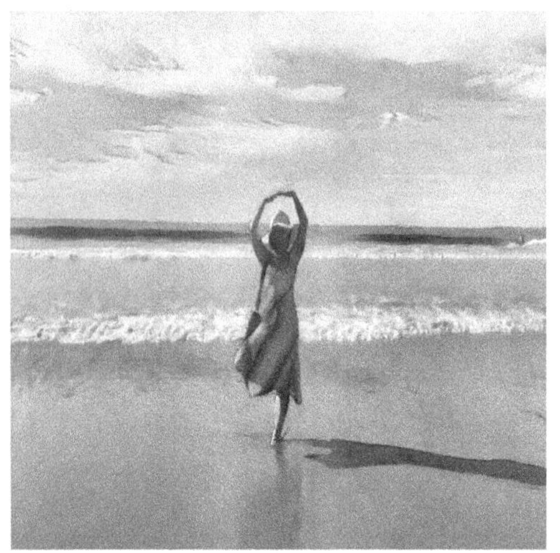 as I recover". But later the hospital discovers Garcia is

infected with Covid-19. When Natalia learns he has the

virus and he will not be home for Christmas, she is

feeling sad and remembers all the beautiful memories

with him. She feels a lump in her throat and [92]drops of

[93]tears slide down her [94]cheeks. She gets into her car,

goes to the ocean where she used to go with Garcia, and

she looks out at the waves coming into the beach. This song comes to her mind: "Come back and

hold my cold hands again. Don't say goodbye or see my eyes will rain again and again. Waiting

and waiting for you, Darling, darling can't live without you." She remembers their sitting by the

fireplace, he would hold her hands and make them warm.

To lighten the burden of the sadness in her heart, she returns home, and the broken-hearted

Natalia picks up her guitar and starts playing this song for Garcia. She sings the song, posts it on

Facebook and tells everybody this is my Christmas gift to my dear Garcia. Because she sang it

---

[92] a small round-shaped amount of liquid

[93] a drop of salty liquid that flows from the eye, as a result of strong emotion, especially unhappiness, or pain

[94] the soft part of your face that is below your eye

from the bottom of her heart, it touched the hearts of others who heard it on Facebook, and the song went viral.

Section 2: Song and Lyrics: Waiting & Waiting for You

🎧 "Waiting & Waiting for You"

The story of your not being here is sad full of sorrow

Without you there is no way no joy no tomorrow

Come back hold my cold hands again

Don't say goodbye or see my eyes

will rain again and again

Waiting and waiting for you

Darling darling can't live without you

Look, love road is a dead-end without you

No other way, I am so attached to,

I care about you

Without you I am a shattered, broken tree,

So still, so silent waiting for you to reach me

Now it's the new year

It's time, come back to me

Bring your love as a Christmas gift to me

Waiting and waiting for you,

Ah, longing darling darling for you

Section 3: Museum of Reincarnation: Florence Nightingale

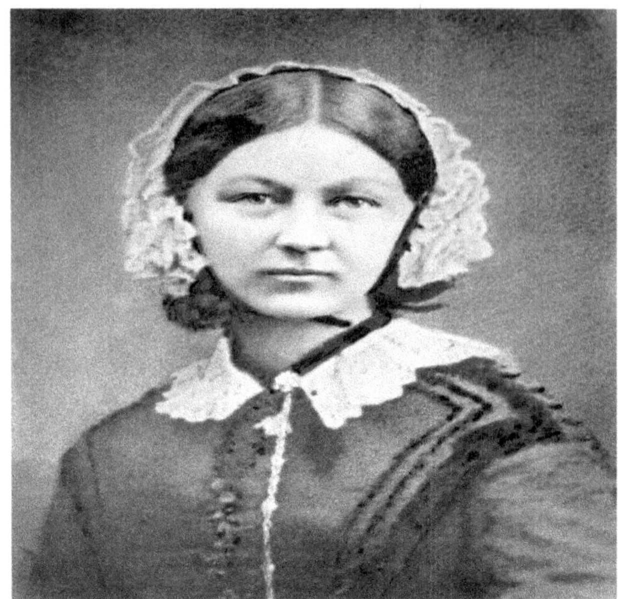

Wikipedia contributors. (2022). *Florence Nightingale.*

🎧 The biography part of the museum (Visit website to listen)

🎧 Visiting the museum (Visit website to watch and listen)

Museum Transcripts

a. Biography

Florence Nightingale (1820 – 1913) was a British [95]social reformer, statistician, and the founder of modern nursing. She [96]came to public attention as a manager and trainer of nurses during the Crimean War. Nightingale organized and cared for wounded soldiers. She was known as the "The Lady with the Lamp," making rounds of wounded soldiers at night. Nightingale was a great and productive writer concerned with spreading [97]medical information. She wrote

---

[95] Social reformer: A person who tries to change the social rules to help people
[96] Came to public attention: Became famous
[97] Medical: related to the treatment of illness and injuries

in simple English so that she could easily be understood by everyone. She was also a leader

in data visualization with the use of infographics, effectively using graphical presentations

of statistical data ("Florence Nightingale.," n.d.). But, most of all, she is famous for her care and

[98]compassion for wounded soldiers. (Reef, C. (2016); Wikipedia contributors, 2022).

Paraphrased Quotations

I took my lamp and medicines to reach wounded soldiers at night. Because I had love and

passion, and I had no fear. There is no way to be successful under the spirit of fear. On your path

to peace, evil appears in different shapes in your life, but you must stay strong and silent when

someone or something contradicts you because then you will learn.

Yes, there is no better definition of a nurse than as a person who cares about patients and is

attached to them. To be blessed, you need to be kind to others. If you only make your own joy,

your pleasure, and not think about others, then you will be destined for eternal damnation" Now,

I am longing to return to the battlefield and be of help to others. I want to say that wise and

humane management of the patient is the best safeguard against any disease.

Paraphrased Quotations taken from Florence Nightingale's quotes on Life, Communication, and

Nursing by Juma, 2020.

Section 4: Deepening our Cultural Understanding: 2019-20 Covid-19 and Front-line Heroes

"2019-20 Covid-19 and Front-line Heroes who have been as patient and strong as a tree"

The COVID-19 pandemic is an infectious disease resulting in acute respiratory

syndrome. The outbreak was first identified in Wuhan, China, in December 2019. The World

Health Organization declared the outbreak a public health emergency of international concern on

---

[98] kindness

30 January and a pandemic on 11 March. As of 26 May 2020, more than 5.49 million cases of COVID-19 have been reported in more than 188 countries and territories, resulting in more than 346,000 deaths. More than 2.23 million people have recovered from the virus. ("COVID-19 pandemic," n.d.)

The 2019-20 Covid-19 is an enemy of every culture and an invisible serial killer in the world. It has torn apart countless families, shattered economies, and left people in shock and sorrow not only in the US but around the world. People around the world are waiting for the virus to go away. The coronavirus has changed every living culture. We can no longer touch those we love. We stay away from each other. We stay in the house. The virus is the cultural emergency of this century. The virus has caused time to stop as everyone is sheltered in place. The virus is not waiting for us. We are waiting for the virus to go away. Waiting and waiting at home and depending upon technology are everybody's culture these days.

The Heroes: Those Who Did Not Wait and Did Help

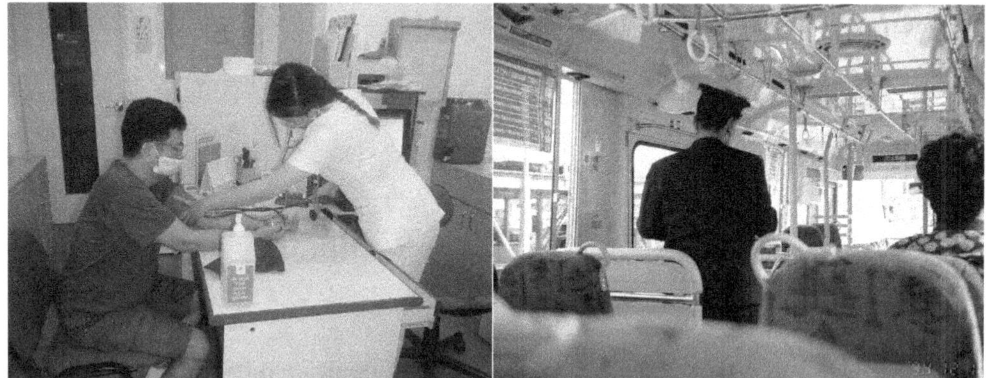

Wikipedia contributors. (2020, June 20)

The nurses in hospitals all around the country are our true heroes. They are the ones who are not waiting, and instead, they are fighting the virus. They get up each day and report to hospitals that are struggling to provide care to the victims of the covid-19 virus. These nurses are putting their health and safety on the line each day as they provide the primary care for those who are suffering. Nurses around the country report the same concerns and fears. They are working long hours and experience the fear of not knowing if they are going to be infected. They care for the dying whose families cannot be with them. Nurses have to hold the hands of the dying. Of course, they console the families and comfort them as best they can. At the end of the day, they go home and shower in the basement, and change clothes before going upstairs to be with their families. They are encouraged by the kindness shown to them by friends and neighbors who bring food and drinks and leave it at their doorsteps. The restaurants deliver meals on the weekends. The kindness of strangers is everywhere. Being kinder is everybody's culture these days.

Bus drivers, transit workers, firemen and policewomen, and men are also putting their health and lives on the line as they provide the essential services that make life in our cities and towns possible. Each day these public servants leave their families and go out to serve others. Despite the pandemic, they report to work each day to repair the buses, and trains, clean the stations and buses and report to the firehouses and police stations so that life can go on in the cities. Hundreds of these essential workers have lost their lives in cities large and small. The covid-19 virus has impacted these workers more than most, and many of these workers are people of color. The virus has had a very large impact on communities of color. This large impact on communities of color is causing a renewed conversation about the need to provide the health services necessary to keep all our citizens healthy and well. They have been strong and patient heroes and a source of strength like the trees.

Celebrities Who Celebrated First Responders and Nurses

"The stars take part in One World: Together at Home concert: Some of the biggest names in music have joined forces to celebrate healthcare workers in a globally televised concert. Lady

Gaga, Paul McCartney, and Billie Eilish were among more than 100 artists who performed songs from their living rooms due to the coronavirus lockdown. The Rolling Stones even managed to play together from four separate locations. The eight-hour show also featured real-life stories from those on the front line of the fight against the Covid-19 virus. The event raised almost $128m (£102m), with proceeds going towards vaccine development and local and regional charities, Organizers Global Citizen said. Lady Gaga, who curated the line-up, called the event "a love letter to the world". Dedicating the show to first responders and medical staff, she said the participating musicians all wanted "to give back a little bit of the kindness that you've given us" (Savage, 2020).

Section 5: Yoga Posture: Tree

Yoga Posture: Tree (Asana: Virkshasana)
Virksha: Tree; Asana: posture

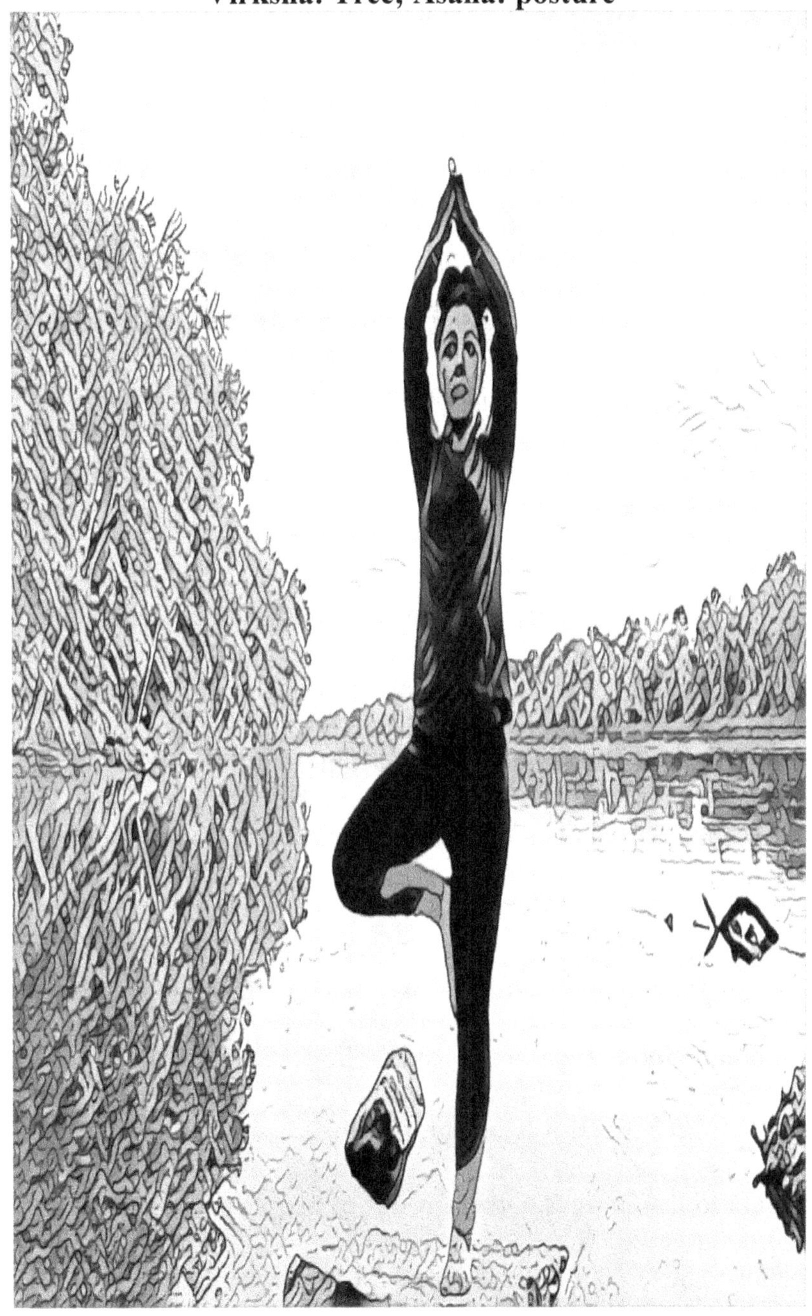

When you are overwhelmed by the difficulties in life, just be patient and strong like an oak tree and believe that the spring of your life is on its way!

Mythology of Virkshasana

"In many Indian traditions, trees are symbols of love and devotion. Many native cultures seek the knowledge of trees for healing, searching their branches, trunks, leaves, and roots for powerful medicines. Patient by nature, trees are quiet and steady, living their long lives in rhythm with the seasons and the circadian rhythm of the world. Trees often appear as sacred symbols of the universe, a bridge between the creator and the individual" (Gaia, 2018). Because of its hollow center, bamboo is resilient and less susceptible to breakage. It can bend but not break. To the Chinese, this characteristic corresponds with the ideals of a Confucian scholar - strong yet modest and flexible.

The tree pose offers a beautiful opportunity to meditate on a tree's inherent qualities. The tree is so tolerant that it even gives shade to the woodcutter, who comes to cut it down with an ax. The true yogi freely gives the fruits of spiritual wisdom and love as generously as trees. Trees tolerate all kinds of natural disturbances, torrents of rain, scorching heat, and piercing cold. The tree pose is a posture in which we give body, mind, and breath the qualities of generosity, forbearance, strength, and balance (Kaivalya, 2016).

Every part of the globe has a myth about trees. From the oak in central Europe, ash in Scandinavia, and Shorea in India, trees are revered. They cultivated and protected holy trees and would beg forgiveness from a tree if it were cut. In Korea, spirits of women who died in childbirth were thought to live in trees. Other groups of people considered trees tightly bound with their own creation. The Greeks believed the first man was made from an ash tree. In Siberia, man and woman were thought to have been created separately from a larch and a fir. Scandinavian myths state gods breathed life into two tree trunks to make the first human couple. Other northern Europeans believed man was first carved from an alder. In Indonesia, vertical slices cut into a fig tree by two gods created man, while horizontal slices created woman. In New Guinea, man was considered a tree that moved! Some trees were well known for their special attributes. In many areas, birch was the tree of health, wisdom, and safety -- used in baby cradles and cribs and used as symbols of public office. Cedars were the trees of paradise in the Mideast. They were also symbols of faithful lovers in China and were held as sacred in Nepal. Junipers were planted as protection from thieves and witches (Coder, 2011).

Connection to the lesson

In this period of her life, Natalia is so sad because Garcia, who is the love of her life, is diagnosed with a bad virus in China. She is trying to be patient, and in order to create a balance in her feelings, she writes a song and expresses her feeling to Garcia. She is trying to be strong and patient as a tree.

Cautionary notes

- Do not raise your arms, if you have heart issues.

- Keep your toes on the ground if it's difficult for you to keep your balance.

- Ensure your knees are soft if you have discomfort in your knees.

Yogic Breathing: Dirgha Pranayama

Meaning: Prana: air; life force; Yama: to restrain or hold back

Potential effects

Enhancement of complete and full breathing, decreasing stress and tension while calming the mind and the body, helping the lungs remain healthy by increasing the oxygen flow to the blood, it massages the abdominal organs, facilitating digestion, preparing you for a better learning experience.

Three Breathing Steps: (Visit website to listen)

1- Sit up straight with your shoulders back and down with relaxed abdominals.

2- Relax the face, close your mouth, and place your hands on your belly.

3- Breathe into your belly and feel it expands like a balloon. Repeat several times.

4- Now, put your hands to the sides of your rib cage and breathe into them, feeling the rib cage expand, and repeat several times.

5- Put your fingertips on your upper chest. Breathe into it and feel your hands lifting. Repeat several times.

6- Now, make a complete inhalation. As you are inhaling, feel the expansions of your belly, rib cage, and chest, and as you are exhaling, you feel the contractions of all three. Repeat this series several times (Refer to Figure 1 in Chapter 1).

Next, move into the warmup, which is the next section.

Warm up: Standing Hip Circles (To listen click here)

Stand tall with your feet about shoulder-width apart and place your hands on your hips. Ensure that your knees are not locked, start to move your hips in a circle. Inhale and exhale, and little by little, make the circles larger and larger (Figure 1).

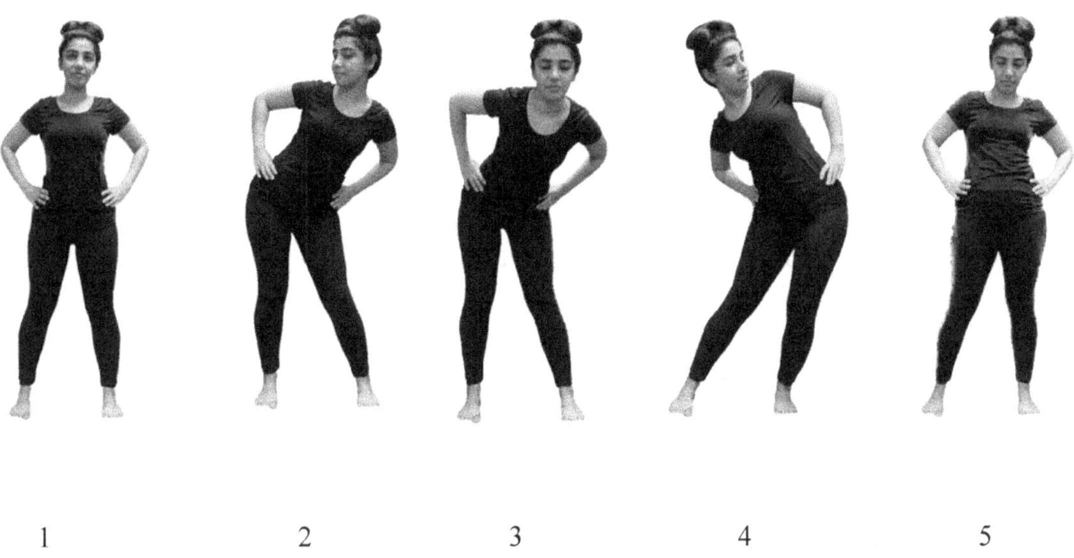

1   2   3   4   5

Figure 1: Standing Hip Circles

Posturer steps of Tree (Virkshasana): (Visit website to listen)

1- Stand tall with your feet hip-width apart, inhale and transfer your weight onto your left foot.

2- On an inhale, raise your right foot as high as is comfortable. While keeping your balance and breathing deeply, grasp your right foot and place it on the inside of your left thigh. (If you have difficulty putting your right foot on your left thigh, then lean your foot on the inside of your ankle).

3- On an inhale, raise your arms to the sides, palms facing forward. Keep your abs active and lengthen your back.

4- Inhale as you are rooting yourself through the standing leg, exhale and lift your arms and stretch toward the sky. Soften your shoulders, move them back and down and straighten your back. Gaze at a spot on the ground and maintain your balance. Hold the pose for a few seconds.

5-   To release, on an exhale, bring your arms down by your side and then lower your raised leg down to the ground.

6-   Relax and feel the difference of Virkshasana (tree pose) and repeat with the right leg (Figure 2).

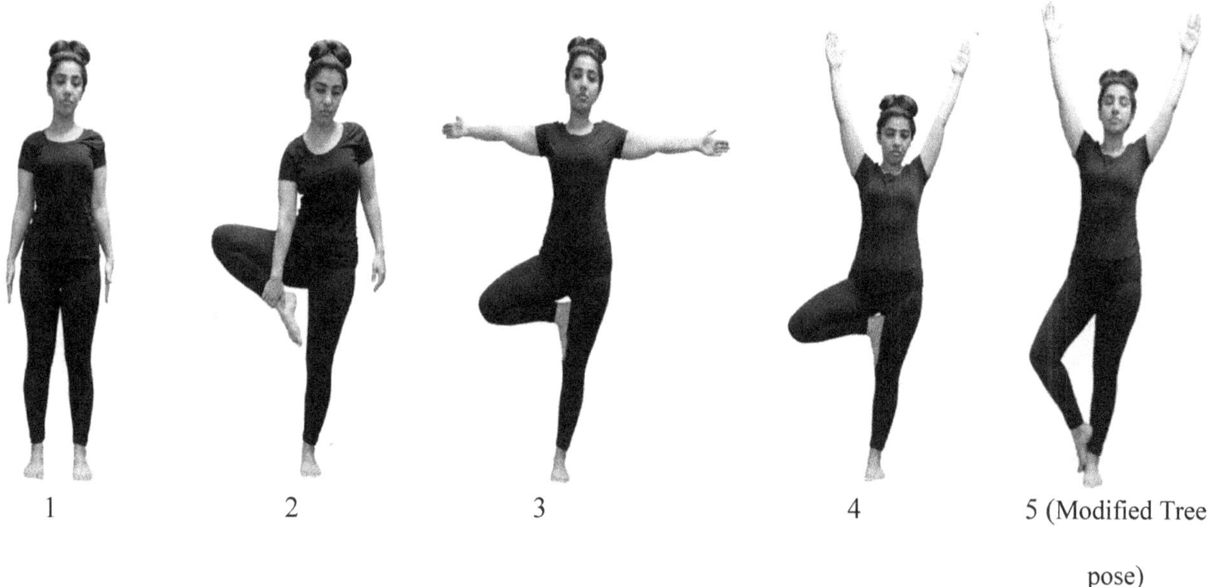

Figure 2: Tree (Virkshasana)

Chapter 6

Section 1: Short Story: Liar

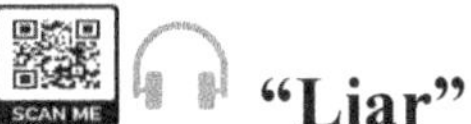 **"Liar"**

Four months have passed, and Garcia has not returned from China. Garcia and Natalia have been in communication through WhatsApp and FaceTime. Slowly Garcia has become less interested in talking to Natalia. One day Natalia is browsing Facebook, and suddenly she sees pictures of Garcia taken from an English language newspaper in China. It is a story of a young

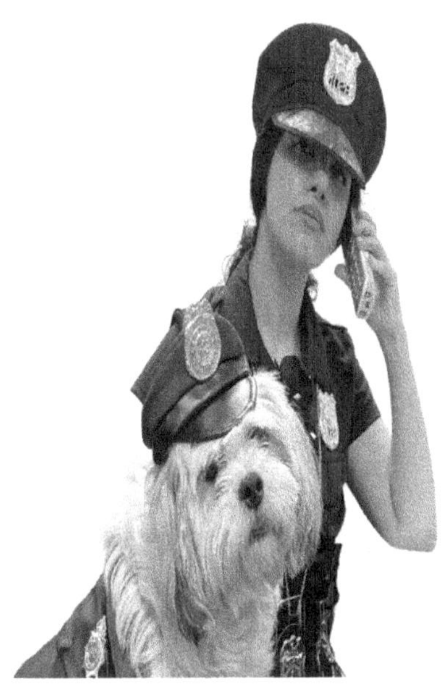

businessman from America who has fallen in love with his Chinese nurse. The story received a lot of likes on Facebook because of the reversed and positive effects of Covid-19. Natalia is UMSSAD (upset, mad, sad, shocked, angry, and disappointed). She does not know what to do. Three months have passed, and she has been trying to get in touch with Garcia, but no reply from him. At that time, she receives a private Facebook message sent by Li, the Chinese nurse, who befriended

Garcia in China. The nurse explains that she listened to the "Waiting and Waiting" song that Natalia sang on Facebook, and she loved the lyrics and discovered that it was a gift to Garcia. Then she explains how hurt and devastated she was because Garcia betrayed her too. He promised to marry her, took her money, and disappeared.

When Natalia hears the story from the Chinese nurse, she becomes angry, but she tries to stay strong and put her anger aside. She starts to find her way to become a warrior. She begins to think critically and asks the following questions: "Who can help me? How can I get justice? Why did this happen to me? When and where did I make a mistake? Should I call 911?". She sits down, talks to her dad, and tells him the whole story. Her dad is so supportive and tells her "I am sorry daughter that this jerk hurt you. I will do everything to support you."

They recognized that Garcia is a criminal who has betrayed Natalia and the nurse in China. They decided to call the police because Natalia wants justice. She calls 911 and tells the police that she has been swindled and she knows of at least one other woman who has been swindled by Garcia. When Garcia returns from Wuhan to Logan International Airport, he is immediately arrested by the police. Now he is in prison and waiting for his trial.

Section 2: Song and Lyrics: Liar

"Liar"

I wonder what what are the reasons

for all your treasons

I wonder why, why

you told me lie

I wonder how how

You dumped me why, tell me now why

Tell me now why, you dumped me how

Gotta know who who

love you the way I do

Tell me now when when

when your betrayals begin?

I wonder where where

maybe now I should not care

I'm gonna say goodbye

Do you wanna know why why

Cause this love is dead

It's too late

Alll I have now is a headache

Now I wanna call 911

It's all over I am all done

SOS help help 911

He has cheated me lied to me it's over I am done

I got a phobia from his lies

Do something for me guys

911 my heart is on fire

It's burning he is a liar

Wanted wanted by police

These lies have surely got to cease

This liar looks cute and chic

But he's nothing except slick

this liar is now in prison

Because of his lies and treasons

Section 3: Museum of Reincarnation: Hatshepsut

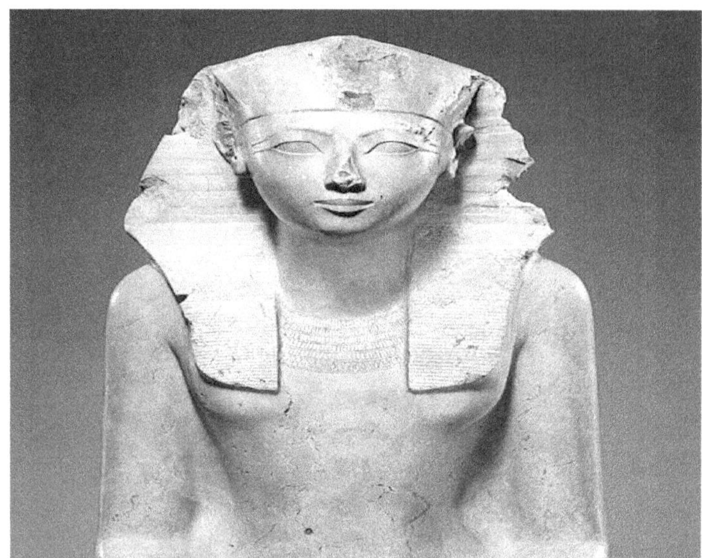

Wikipedia contributors. *Hatshepsut*

Museum Transcripts

🎧 The biography part of the museum (Visit website to listen)

🎧 Visiting the museum (Visit website to watch and listen)

a. Biography

Hatshepsut (1507–1458 BC) was the fifth [99]pharaoh of the Eighteenth Dynasty of Egypt.

she was the longest-reigning female pharaoh in Egypt, ruling for 20 years in the 15th century

B.C. She is considered one of the most successful pharaohs.

According to American [100]archeologist and Egyptologist James Henry Breasted, she is also

known as "the first great woman in the history of whom we are informed." Under her reign,

---

[99] (The title of) a king of ancient Egypt
[100] someone who studies the buildings, graves, tools, and other objects of people who lived in the past

Egypt [101]prospered. she was more interested in ensuring economic prosperity and building and restoring [102]monuments throughout Egypt rather than in [103]conquering new lands.

An attempt was made to remove all traces of Hatshepsut's rule. Her statues were torn down, her monuments were defaced, and her name was removed from the official king's list (Green, 2014). Why was the history of Hatshepsut's reign erased from Egyptian history? The reason for her removal was the fact that she was a woman. Her success was against the traditions of male supremacy.

b. Paraphrased Quotations

"I wonder why the men of my land could not accept the rule of a woman?" "You got to know I was a woman warrior" "When they destroyed my statues, they lied to the world about history. It was a betrayal to the world. No doubt that those guys committed treasons. I wanna show the truth to the world. Destroying and burning my statues does not burn my heart and my soul because "I have done things according to the design of my heart." Put aside your phobias and fears. Women are leaders, too. "I have commanded that my title abide like the mountains; when the sun shines, its rays shine brightly upon my majesty;" I don't care that "my name was removed from the official king list" because now my good work is shining in the history of the world. I am not dead; you destroyed my statue and everything except my majesty. I don't know what the future holds, and I wonder if people will one day understand women are the equals of men. Quotes taken from Hatshepsut, wikiquotes.

---

[101] Became successful
[102] a structure or building that is built to honor a special person or event
[103] Taking control

Section 4: Deepening our Cultural Understanding: Critical Thinking and Feeling of Justice

Definition of lying: It is a clear decision made by a person to not tell the truth. All cultures and religions value honesty. Every culture judges lying as being wrong and truth as right.

Garcia is a liar! He made a choice not to tell Natalia the truth. Garcia did two things wrong: he lied to Natalia, and he also took her money. Lying is wrong and immoral. Taking her money is also immoral and a crime punishable by a jail sentence.

How do we know that someone is lying and immoral? An immoral act is an act that a culture agrees is wrong.

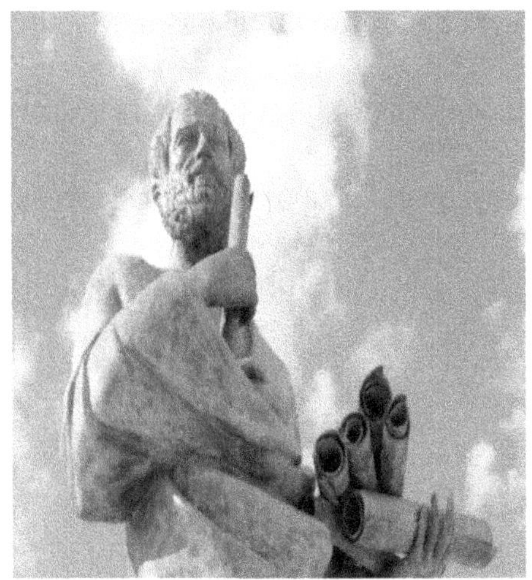

The Greek philosopher, Aristotle, gave us a way of telling right from wrong. You can tell if something is right or wrong by the feeling. You should ask yourself, "Is this right or wrong?"; Life is complicated, and Aristotle devised critical thinking questions to help us decide if an act is right or wrong. His critical thinking questions were: (what happened, who did it, when, where, how, and why?); Over the centuries, these questions were adopted by the courts to determine if the testimony was truthful. If you ask the question why, what happened, who, where, when, and how the action was performed, we have enough information to judge if the person is telling the truth.

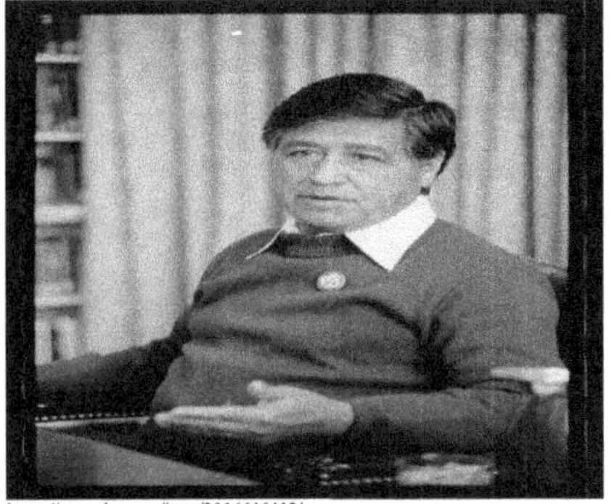
https://www.loc.gov/item/2016646413/

Cesar Estrada Chavez (1927-1993)

The civil rights leader Cezar Chavez says that right and wrong are something that you can see and feel. When he saw agricultural workers doing backbreaking work in the sun for low wages and no health care, he knew this was wrong.

Cesar Chavez is a critical cultural thinker who was a labor organizer, a leader, and a civil rights activist who transformed the lives and opportunities of tens of thousands of Mexican and Mexican American agricultural workers who labored in the fields of the west, southwest, and throughout the United States. Agricultural labor is backbreaking, hot, dirty work performed by immigrants and poor people. Cesar was introduced to injustice at a young age when his father was swindled out of the family land, and the family was forced to move from Yuma, Arizona, to San Jose, California. When his dad was injured in an auto accident, Cesar quit school and went to work in the grape vineyards. He was UMSSAD at the conditions in the fields, and he set out to organize the workers to get better wages and working conditions. His work was groundbreaking because no one had dared to organize agricultural workers before. After much struggle, he was successful, and today farm workers have much improved wages and working conditions because of this courageous and determined leader.

Cesar Chavez gives us a different way of critical thinking. He looked at the world, and he trusted his feelings to tell him right from wrong. Like Cesar Chavez, you can trust your feelings and your ability to tell right from wrong.

Section 5: Yoga Posture: Warrior

Yoga Posture: Warrior (Asana: Virabhadrasana)
Vira: bravery, courage; Bhadra: blessed, auspicious; Asana: Posture

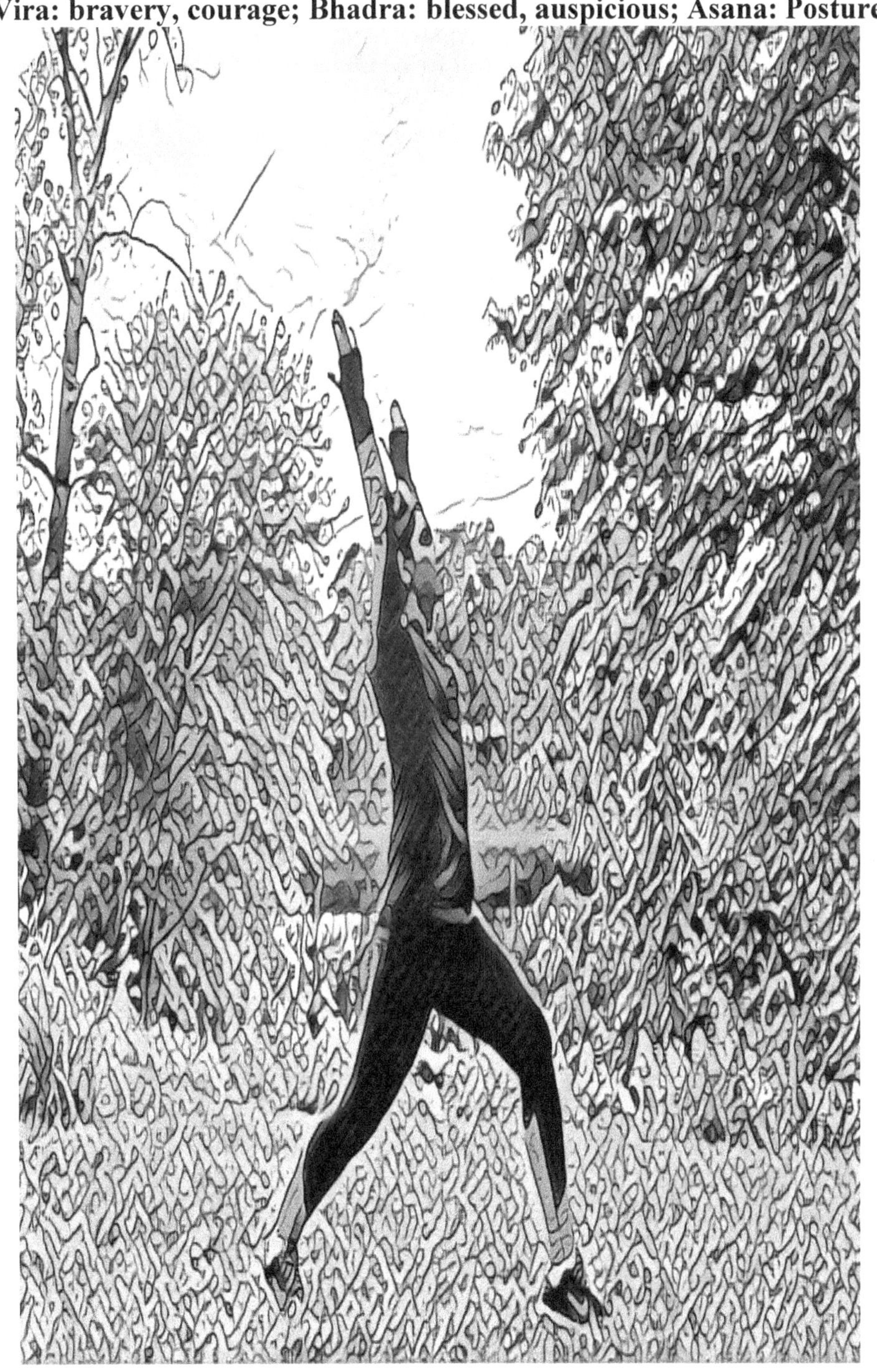

When the lies, fear and negative energies in life find their way into your head and discourage you, do not give up. Turn it around, fight back, defeat them and show them you are a warrior!

Mythology of Virabhadrasana

This glorious standing pose is taken from the great hero warrior Virabhadra from Hindu mythology. This is an active posture that requires strength, steadiness, and a fierce determination to hold with integrity. We practice this pose not to condone violence but to honor our fight against our own ignorance and ego and to cultivate strength and courage to do the right thing under difficult circumstances.

The warrior Virabhadra was created by Shiva, one of the major Hindu Gods, to avenge the death of his beloved wife, Sati. Daksha, Sati's father, did not approve of her marriage to Shiva, so when Daksha decided to hold a huge festival, he did not invite Shiva or Sati. Sati was hurt by this snub and her father's refusal to accept her marriage, and she decided to go to the festival and confront him. Daksha asked why she was there since she was not invited, and he rudely asked if she had finally come to her senses and left that "wild animal of a husband." Sati was saddened and humiliated and decided to end her own life, not wanting to be associated with her father anymore. She throws herself into the sacrificial fires of the festival, and her body bursts into flames. When Shiva heard the news of his wife's death, he was at first devastated, then enraged. In a fury, he tore out one of his dreadlocks and threw it to the ground. Virabhadra was created, springing up from the energy released by the ferociously thrown dreadlock. "*Vira*" means "Hero," and "*Bhadra*" means "Auspicious." Virabhadrasana (Warrior) represents Virabhadra as he emerges up from under the ground, arms reaching up and gazing upwards (Karen, H.C, 2015).

Connections to the lesson

In this Part, Natalia feels devastated when she finds out about Garcia's lies, but she never gives up, and she starts to do some critical thinking (asking Aristotle's WH questions) and fighting not to repeat past mistakes. In this chapter, the author likens Natalia's personality to Virabhadrasana (Warrior), which represents Virabhadra as he emerges up from under the ground, arms reaching up, holding the critical thinking ball, and gazing upwards. Natalia gets angry and talks to her father. Then she is ready to fight. She calls the police to take her rights back.

Cautionary notes

- If you have a persistent circulatory or heart issue or high/low blood pressure, please consult your physicians.

- Avoid holding the posture for a long period of time, and do not raise your hands above your shoulder.

Yogic Breathing: Dirgha Pranayama

Meaning: Prana: air; life force; Yama: to restrain or hold back

Potential effects

Enhancement of complete and full breathing, decreasing stress and tension while calming the mind and the body, helping the lungs remain healthy by increasing the oxygen flow to the blood, it massages the abdominal organs, facilitating digestion, preparing you for a better learning experience.

Three Breathing Steps: (Visit website to listen)

1- Sit up straight with your shoulders back and down with relaxed abdominals.

2- Relax the face, close your mouth, and place your hands on your belly.

3- Breathe into your belly and feel it expands like a balloon. Repeat several times.

4- Now, put your hands to the sides of your rib cage and breathe into them, feeling the rib cage expand, and repeat several times.

5- Put your fingertips on your upper chest. Breathe into it and feel your hands lifting. Repeat several times.

6- Now, make a complete inhalation. As you are inhaling, feel the expansions of your belly, rib cage, and chest, and as you are exhaling, you feel the contractions of all three. Repeat this series several times (Refer to Figure 1 in Chapter 1).

Next, move into the warmup, which is the next section.

🎧 Warm-up: Standing Lunge (Visit website to listen)

- Stand tall with your feet hip-width apart. Keep your torso long and straight. Soften your shoulders back and down.

- On an inhale, step forward with one leg, lowering your hips until both knees are bent at about a 90-degree angle. Your front knee should be above your ankle. Do not let your back knee touch the floor. Keep the weight on your heels as you push back up to the starting position. Rest and try it on the other side (Figure 1).

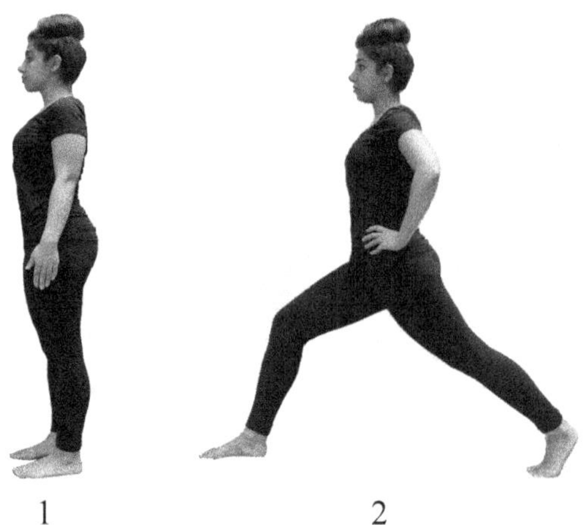

1   2

Figure 1: Standing Lung

Posture steps for Warrior (Virabhadrasana): **(Visit website to listen)**

1- Stand tall with your feet hip-width apart.

2- Inhale, and as you exhale, step back with your left foot, about 3 to 4 feet. Bend your right knee and lower your hips. Be sure that the knee is stacked directly over the ankle. Align your feet so that they are hip-width apart.

3- Square your hips and, on an inhale, lengthen your waist and raise your arms up to the sky into a V position. Roll your shoulders back and down and arch your upper back slightly. Ensure that your neck is aligned with the rest of your back. Hold the pose for a few seconds.

4- To release, on an exhale, lower your arms and step forward. Feel the difference of Virabadrasana/the Warrior pose and repeat on the other side (Figure 2).

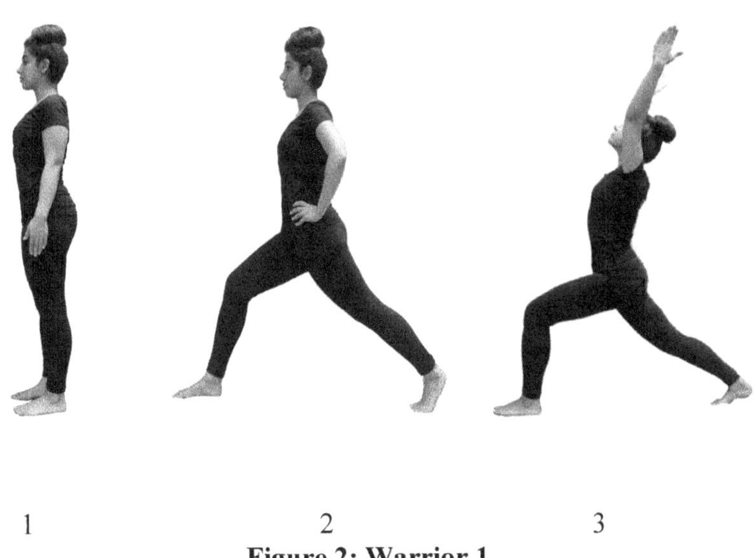

1   2   3

Figure 2: Warrior 1

Chapter 7

Section 1: Short Story: Becoming a Fighter

 **"Becoming a Fighter"**

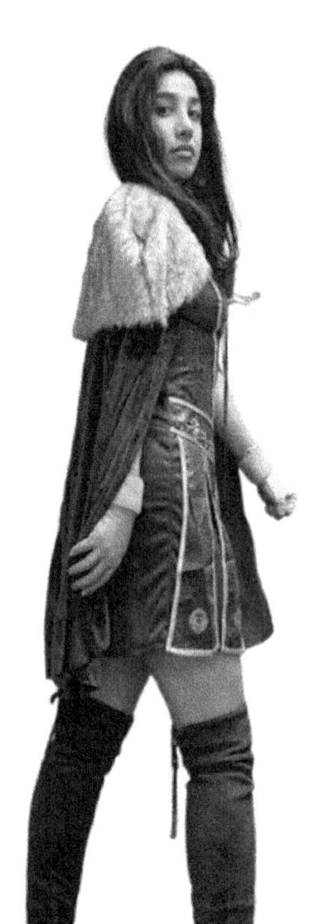

While Garcia is in prison waiting for his trial, Natalia is still UMSSAD (upset, mad, sad, shocked, angry, and disappointed). She was running away from what she does not know, and what she cannot control. One night, It is raining, it is pouring. Suddenly she wakes up at 2:00 o'clock in the morning. She has a scary dream, and her heart is racing. She thinks to herself "my life is changing". She rushes to her desk to get her notebook and writes down what is on her mind. She writes: "I am an insomniac and a maniac listening to the rain drops on the rooftop." A picture comes into her mind. She is running from fear. Suddenly she stops and faces her fear. She is not afraid of failure anymore. Fear caused her to panic. She continues writing: "no point in crying, and there is no denying, this is a new beginning. I will face my fear. I am a warrior.

She decides to face her demons, she will tell the story that she was in love with a man who cheated her and took her money. She creates a Facebook Page and shares her story with the world. The other women who were deceived by the Garcias in the world joined her page and posted their stories. Her Facebook page becomes famous because she has started a movement in which women can face their fears, tell their stories of being deceived, harassed, taken advantage of, and fighting back.

A month later, Garcia's trial takes place. Natalia is the first witness. She tells her story and when she finishes, she turns to Garcia and says: "I told you my heart is tender, and my mind is tough". Next, Li; the Chinese woman comes forward to tell her story. Garcia pleads guilty and goes to jail for a long time and the judge returns Li and Natalia's money plus the damages for the suffering they have experienced.

Now Natalia is a stronger, she is fighting hard to educate women about their rights, she has returned to college and now she is majoring in women's studies. One day while walking on campus, she happens to meet Sam, her high school crush. Now all the memories come flooding back about the moon.

To be continued….

Section 2: Song and Lyrics: Becoming a Fighter

"Becoming a Fighter"

Tonight, it's pouring , it's raining

I feel like life is changing

I am listening to raindrops

Sliding on our rooftop

Tonight, I am an insomniac

I am a maniac

Sound of clock ticking

The fast heart beating

"Time is flying

No point in crying

No point in denying

"This is a new beginning

A feeling of winning

The heart is debating

I am done with waiting" (2)

Just like a volcano

Ready to erupt you know

can't put out this brutal fire

can't forget my wild desire

Tonight, I can't help thinking

My damn mind is freaking

My beating heart is racing

My crazy thoughts are chasing

Tonight, I'm an insomniac

I am a maniac

Sound of clock ticking

The fast heart beating

I am a survivor

Who is still a fighter

I can break all the barriers

I am a warrior (2)

Section 3: Museum of Reincarnation: Albert Einstein

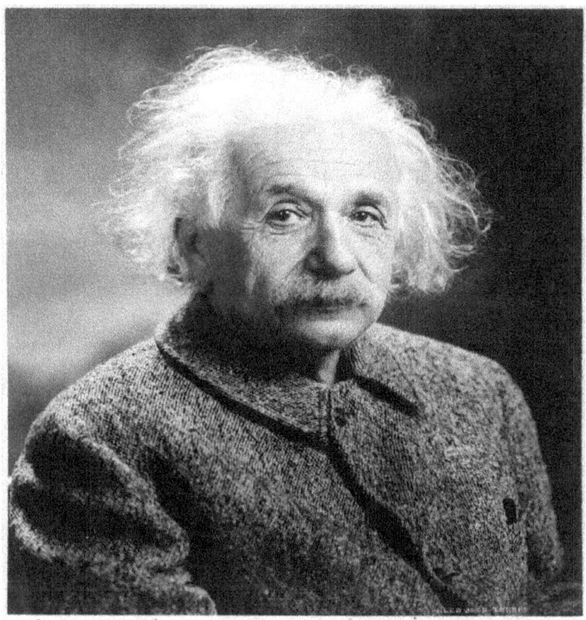

Turner O.J. (1947). Albert Einstein.

🎧 The biography part of the museum (Visit website to listen)

🎧 Visiting the museum (Visit website to watch and listen)

Museum Transcripts

a. Biography

Albert Einstein (1879-1965), born in Germany, was one of the great physicists of all time. His theory of relativity is one of the foundations of modern physics. The theory of Relativity is a picture and explains how the objects in the sky, earth, and the universe are related to each other using the laws of physics. The other foundation of physics is Quantum theory which is a picture of the sub-atomic world. Cause and effect are different in the quantum world. An element can be in two places at the same time. Now, how weird is that? The quantum world is a different place with different laws. A Munich schoolmaster wrote in Albert Einstein's school report, "He will never amount to anything," 1895., but he became everything in the world of physics ("Albert Einstein.," n.d. Neffe, J. (2007); Isaacson, W. (2007); Wikipedia contributors (2022).

b. Paraphrased Quotations

I finished my training as a physicist, and the only position I could find was as a clerk in the patent office. There were a lot of problems, but I learned we could not solve our problems with the same thoughts we used when we created them. This was one of the low points of my life and this was the time that I wrote the general theory of relativity, the publication that made me famous. Critical thinking can make you a survivor. When I was a young man hopes and striving were chasing me. Later, I realized we should not limit ourselves to our personal desires. We must free ourselves to embrace compassion for everybody and everything. We need to have great spirits to solve problems. Few are those who can see with their own eyes and feel with their heart beating. However, great spirits have always encountered wild and brutal opposition from mediocre minds, you need to be a fighter, and my last advice is when you are done with your share, leave elegantly. (Albert Einstein Quotes. (n.d.). BrainyQuote.com. Retrieved June 6, 2020; Button, S. (2017); Goodread. (2020)).

Section 4: Deepening our Cultural Understanding: Fighter Women from History

"Beyond Wonder Woman: Mighty Female Warriors"

While the woman in the 2017 movie "Wonder Woman" is fictional, she has no [104]shortage of

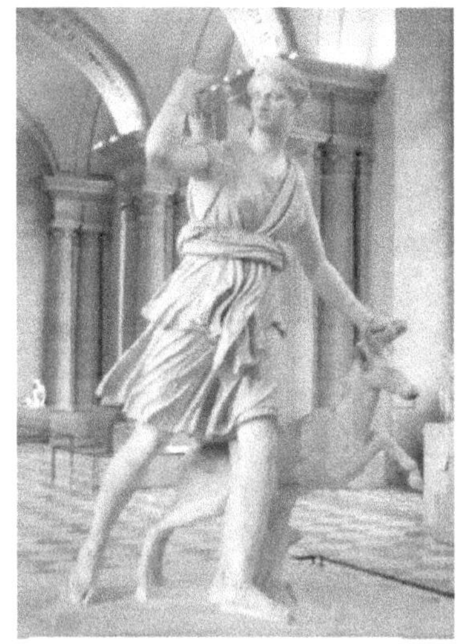

real-world [105]precedents. Throughout history and across cultures, women have been warriors, leading armies of both men and women, proving themselves to be great fighters and highly skilled leaders. (Weisberger, 2017)

"[106]"Fu Hao is the earliest known female general from the Shang Dynasty who lived about 3,000 years ago. More than 100 weapons were found buried in her tomb, confirming her status as a high-

ranking military leader". Boudicca, a fierce military leader, led a tribe from eastern Britain in an

uprising against interlopers during the Roman invasion and occupation of southern England in

the first century. [107]"Ethiopia was once ruled by [108] Queen Gudit."[109]Tomoe Gozen, legendary

female Japanese military leader, was described as a skilled archer. Ana Nzinga ascended to rule

as queen of Ndonga, an African state in what is now Angola, in 1624.[110] Nachiyar, who is the

first Tamil woman to take up arms against British colonialism in India, grew up in South India,

where she learned as a child to use weapons, practice martial arts, shoot a bow, and fight while

on horseback. Bastidas was born in Peru; In 1780, when her husband Tupac led what would be a

---

[104] lack

[105] history

[106] according to the British Museum

[107] according to a study published in 2000 in the journal Bulletin of the School of Oriental and African Studies

[108] (circa 10th century A.D.)

[109] (circa 1157 – 1247)

[110] (1730 – 1796)

pivotal rebellion against the Spanish, she played an equal part in the uprising, according to historian Charles F. Walker in his [111]book." (Weisberger, 2017)

Atusa Shahbanu, the Empress of the Persian Achaemenid Empire [112]and daughter of Cyrus the Great, was the director of palace affairs. She had a say in deciding who would be sent on military missions. Artemis, another woman warrior, also joined the Persian Navy as a young woman. In her most renowned and recorded battle, the Battle of Salamis[113], she fought against the Greeks for King Xerxes. (Historical women, 2020).

Two Present Day fighters

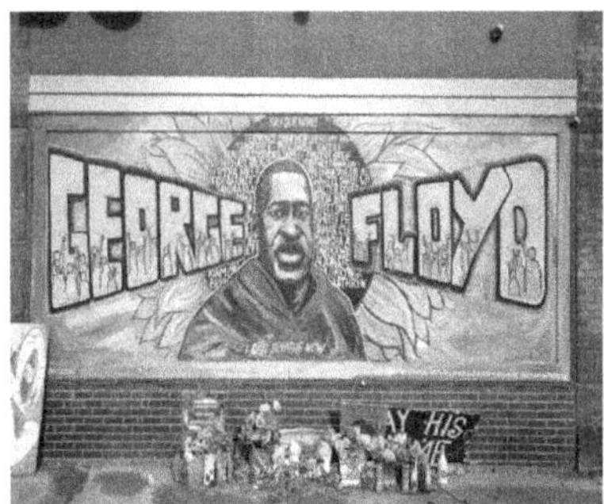

Highsmith, C. M., (2021). George Floyd

George Floyd. (October 14, 1973 – May 25, 2020) died in police [114]custody in Minneapolis, Minn. Mr. Floyd died from [115]asphyxiation due to a [116]chokehold in which a policeman held a knee upon his throat for 8 minutes and forty-two seconds. This [117]horrific scene was videotaped; the video went viral and left people heartbroken. For the first time, people had a visual picture rather than a verbal description of [118]racial violence. His death created a global culture in which people stood together and fought for racial equality. He brought unity among people across race,

---

[111] "The Tupac Amaru Rebellion" (Harvard University Press, 2016)
[112] (522–486 B.C.E.),
[113] (480 BC)
[114] the state of being kept in prison, especially while waiting to go to court for trial
[115] to cause someone to be unable to breathe, usually resulting in that person's death
[116] a way of holding someone with your arm tightly around their neck so that they cannot breathe easily
[117] very bad and shocking
[118] actions or words related to the race of people that are intended to hurt them

skin color, religion, and nationality. This is the first time in history that people are united in their call for racial equality and an end to police brutality. He is the reason everyone can now breathe the word freedom in unity. The protests have resulted in local, state, and federal changes in policing policies and procedures. In death Mr. Floyd is a global and cultural warrior for racial equality and the "Black Lives Matter" movement.

Charlize Theon

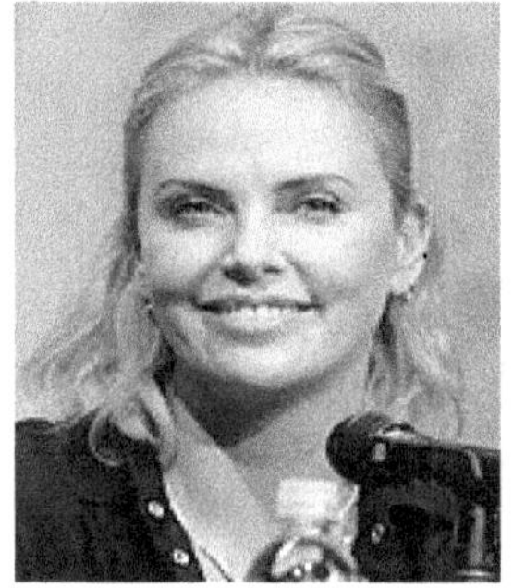

The South African actress was only 15 years old when she [119]witnessed her mother shoot and kill her alcoholic and angry father out of self-defense. But instead of letting that bad experience define her future, she looked to her mother's protective example of strength and worked to build an amazing sense of confidence of her own. She continued to pursue her acting career, and she [120]ultimately became the first South African actress to win an Academy Award." (Hall, 2014).

---

[119] saw
[120] finally

Section 5: Yoga Posture: Side Warrior

Yoga Posture: Side Warrior (Asana: Parshva Virabhadrasana)
Parshva: side; vira: bravery, courage; Bhadra: blessed, auspicious

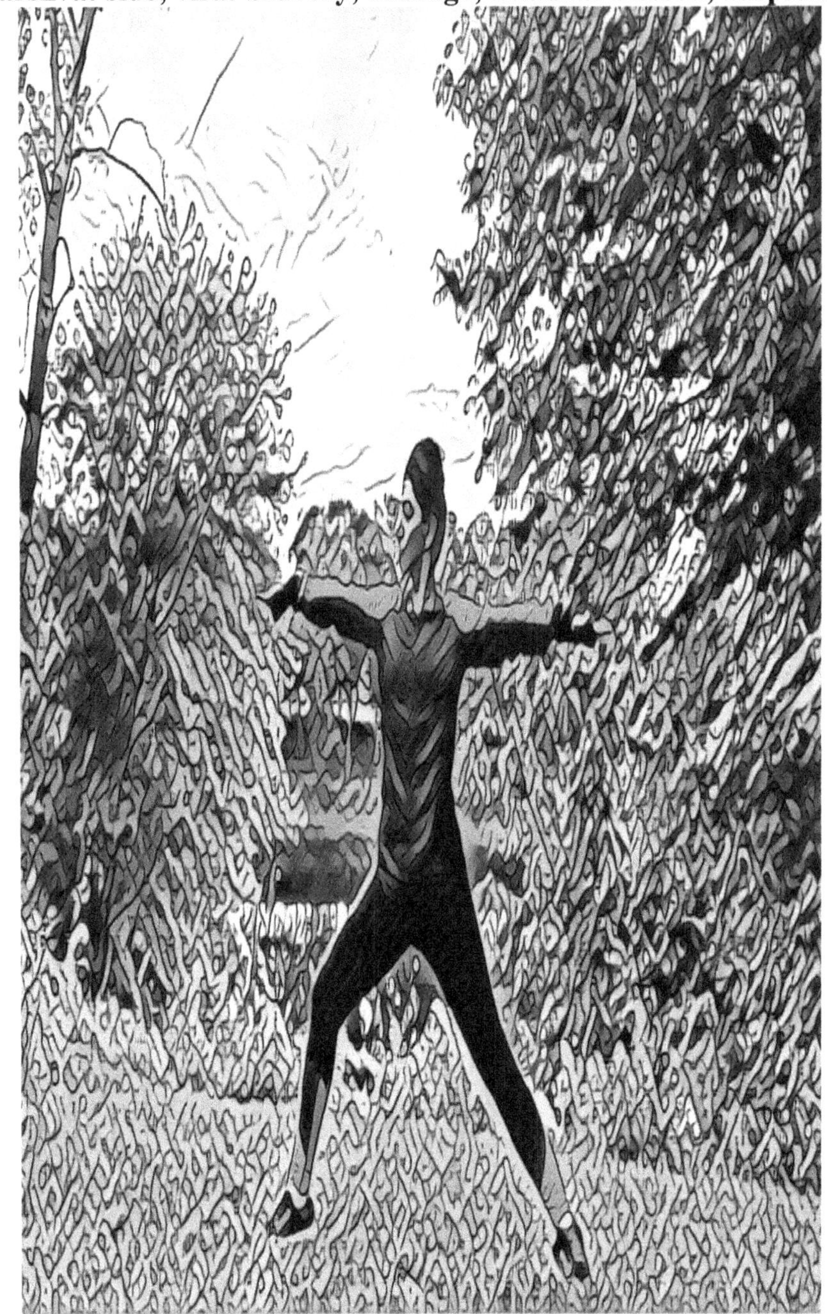

Ride the waves of the difficulties and challenges on the sea of life because the higher the waves are, the greater the opportunities of a critical thinker and warrior to change the world!

Mythology of Parshva Virabhadrasana

In the previous warrior pose, when Shiva heard the news of his wife's death, he was devastated, then enraged. In a fury, he tore out one of his dreadlocks and threw it to the ground. Virabahdra was a huge and terrible being, with a thousand arms, three eyes, and wearing a garland of skulls. Virabhadra sprang from the energy of Shiva's dreadlock. Virabhadra was an angry force that killed all the gods at the festival and cut off Daksha's head. But when Shiva saw the bloody aftermath of this battle, his anger left him. The slain gods were miraculously healed, and Shiva replaced Daksha's head with a goat's head. Daksha and the other gods honored Shiva for this, calling him "Shankar,"," the "kind and benevolent one." Side Warrior portrays when Virabhadra drew his sword and sliced off Daksha's head.

In ancient Iranian mythology, a warrior whose name was Arash was a mighty archer. He lived in those days when the army of the Iranian king Manuchehr was defeated in Mazenderan by the king Turan Afrasiab. The Iranian king wanted to protect the country from the Turanians and made an agreement with Afrasiab. According to the agreement, one of the soldiers had to climb up the mountain of Damavand and shoot an arrow into the sky. The place where the arrow falls will be the border between Turan and Iran. King Afrasiab believed that the arrow would not fly far. Early in the morning, Arash the Archer climbed to the highest point of the mountain, pulled the bow, and shot. He put all his strength and love for his homeland into this arrow, and as soon as he shot the arrow, Arash died. His arrow flew for two days and finally fell next to the Amu Darya River on a land that was far from the Iranian border. Thus, the river became the border between Iran and Turan.

Connection to the lesson

In this chapter, Natalia's love is killed by Garcia. First, she became UMSSAD (upset, mad, sad, shocked, angry, and disappointed), then she overcame the emotional challenges and created a website to fight against the harassment of women. She began to teach other women to be strong like a warrior.

Cautionary notes

- If you have a persistent circulatory or heart issue or high/low blood pressure, please consult your physicians.

- Avoid holding the posture for a long period of time, and do not raise your hands above your shoulder.

Yogic Breathing: Dirgha Pranayama

Meaning: Prana: air; life force; Yama: to restrain or hold back

Potential effects

Enhancement of complete and full breathing, decreasing stress and tension while calming the mind and the body, helping the lungs remain healthy by increasing the oxygen flow to the blood, it massages the abdominal organs, facilitating digestion, preparing you for a better learning experience

Three Breathing Steps

1- Sit up straight with your shoulders back and down with relaxed abdominals.

2- Relax the face, close your mouth, and place your hands on your belly.

3- Breathe into your belly and feel it expands like a balloon. Repeat several times.

4- Now, put your hands to the sides of your rib cage and breathe into them, feeling the rib cage expand, and repeat several times.

5- Put your fingertips on your upper chest. Breathe into it and feel your hands lifting. Repeat several times.

6- Now, make a complete inhalation. As you are inhaling, feel the expansions of your belly, rib cage, and chest, and as you are exhaling, you feel the contractions of all three. Repeat this series several times (Refer to Figure 1 in Chapter 1).

Next, move into the warmup, which is the next section.

Warm-up: Standing Lunge (Visit website to listen)

- Stand tall with your feet hip-width apart. Keep your torso long and straight. Soften your shoulders back and down.

- On an inhale, step forward with one leg, lowering your hips until both knees are bent at about a 90-degree angle. Your front knee should be above your ankle. Do not let your back knee touch the floor. Keep the weight on your heels as you push back up to the starting position. Rest and try it on the other side (Figure 1).

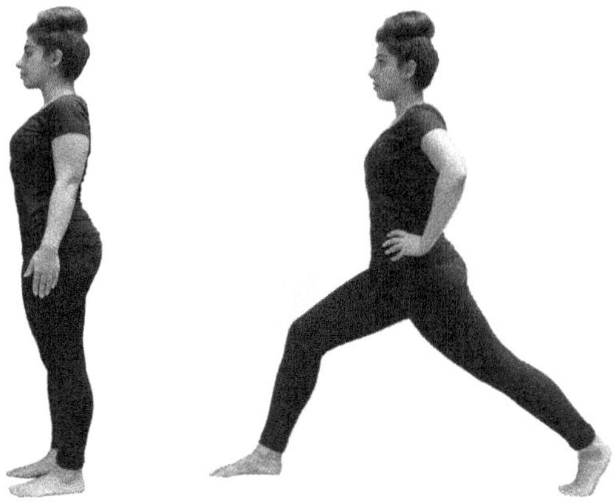

-

1   2

Figure 1: Standing Lung

Posture steps for Side Warrior (Parshva Virabhadrasana): (Visit website to listen)

1- Stand tall in the mountain pose with your feet hip-width apart and your arms by your side.

2- As you are placing your hands on your hips, on an exhale, step back with your right foot, about one leg's length. Bend your left knee and lower your hips.

3- Rotate your back foot and align the arch of your back foot with the sole of your front foot. Level your hips and keep your left knee over your ankle.

4- Breathe deeply. Lengthen your waist and, on an inhale, lift your arms parallel to the floor, palms facing down. Shoulders back and down. Keep your neck straight and look out over your left shoulder. Hold the pose for a few seconds. Keep breathing.

5- To release on an exhale, lower your hands. Square your hips to the front. Exhale and step forward to Tadasana. Rest and feel the effects of Parshva Virabhadrasana. Repeat on the other side (Figure 2).

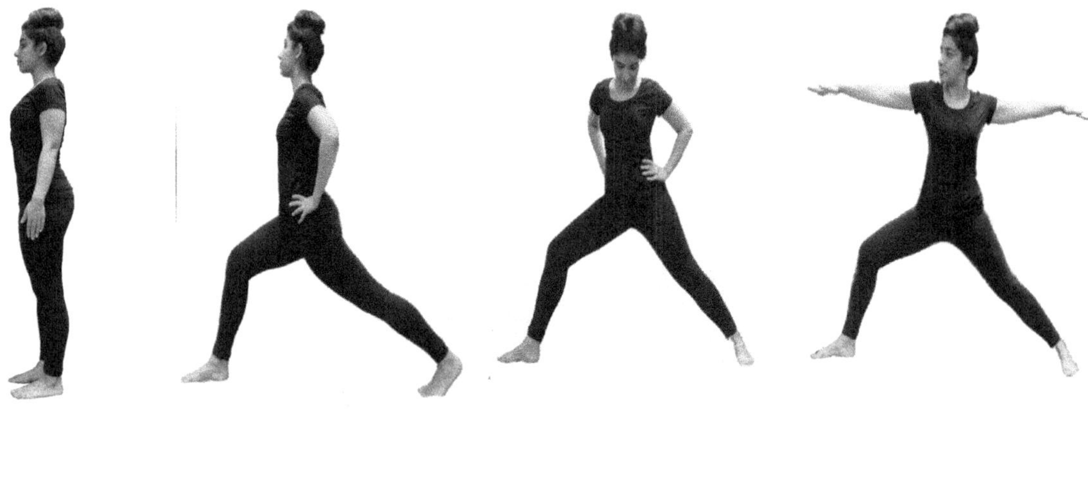

1   2   3   4

Figure 2: Side- Warrior (Parshva-Virabhadrasana)

<u>References</u>

Albert Einstein Quotes. (n.d.). BrainyQuote.com. Retrieved June 6, 2020, from

BrainyQuote.com Website: https://www.brainyquote.com/authors/albert-einstein-quotes

Arslan, G., Yıldırım, M., Zangeneh, M. & AK, I. (2022). Benefits of Positive Psychology-Based

Story Reading on Adolescent Mental Health and Well-Being. *Child Ind Res* 15, 781–793

(2022). https://doi.org/10.1007/s12187-021-09891-4

Bain News Services. P. *Mme. Curie*. Retrieved from the Library of Congress

https://www.loc.gov/pictures/item/2014687674/.

Bedrov, A., & Bulaj, G. (2018). Improving self-esteem with motivational quotes: opportunities

for digital health technologies for people with chronic disorders. *Frontiers in psychology*, *9*,

2126.

Button, S. (2017). *31 Amazing Einstein Quotes On Love, Life and Imagination*. Retrieved from

https://www.spiritbutton.com/albert-einstein-quotes/#ixzz6OpK28HvP

Carson, C. (2001). *The Autobiography of Martin Luther King, Jr.* (Reprint). Warner Books.

Charles River Editors. (2018). *Marie Curie: The Life and Legacy of the Legendary Scientist Who*

Became the First Woman to Win a Nobel Prize. CreateSpace Independent Publishing

Platform.

Coder, K. D. (2011). Cultural aspects of trees: Traditions & myths. Retrieved from

https://athenaeum.libs.uga.edu/bitstream/handle/10724/36443/Cultural%20Aspects%20of%20

Trees%2011-02.pdf?sequence=1

Corliss, J. 2021. Harvard Medical School. https://www.health.harvard.edu/heart-health/yoga-a-

gateway-to-healthier-habits

Czuchry, M., & Dansereau, D. F. (2005). Using motivational activities to facilitate treatment

involvement and reduce risk. *J. Psychoactive Drugs* 37, 7–13. doi:

10.1080/02791072.2005.10399744

Dadvar, A., & Rouzbahani, R. (2016). Role of nature in creation of Iranian Myths. *Asian Social

Science*, *12*(6), 123-131. Retrieved from

https://pdfs.semanticscholar.org/3b3a/39c6d44db6392d088f5753de83c6ccf5b87a.pdf

Ellasar, A.CNN. (2020). Rihanna's foundation donates $5 million to help fight coronavirus.

Retrieved from https://www.cnn.com/2020/03/22/us/rihanna-coronavirus-relief-donation-

trnd/index.html

France, L.R. CNN. (2019). Jennifer Lopez and Alex Rodriguez donate years' worth of food to

Tennessee elementary students. Retrieved from

https://www.cnn.com/2019/10/24/entertainment/jennifer-lopez-alex-rodriguez-donate-

food/index.html

France, L.R. CNN. (2014). Pitbull: 5 surprising facts about the superstar. Retrieved from

https://www.cnn.com/2014/06/20/showbiz/celebrity-news-gossip/pitbull-cnn-

spotlight/index.html

Gaab, N., Schlaug, G., & Wong, L. (2015). Music as Medicine: The impact of healing

harmonies. In *Longwood Seminars* (pp. 1-46).

Gaia. (2018). *Vrksasana: Tree Pose*. Retrieved from https://www.gaia.com/article/vrksasana-

tree-pose

Gardner, H., & Hatch, T. (1989). Educational implications of the theory of multiple

intelligences. *Educational researcher*, *18*(8), 4-10.

Goodread. (2020). Albert Einstein Quotes. Retrieved from

https://www.goodreads.com/quotes/555597-when-i-was-a-fairly-precocious-young-man-i-
became

Green, K. (2014). *The pharaoh that wouldn't be forgotten.* (Hatshepsut) Retrieved from

https://www.youtube.com/watch?v=8bYRy_wZEJI

Hall, A. (2014, August 24). *8 Celebrities Who Transformed Tragedy into Something Positive.*

Retrieved from https://www.huffpost.com/entry/celebrities-overcoming-loss_n_5669363

Highsmith, C. M., photographer. (2021). Hennepin County United States Minnesota

Minneapolis, 2021. -11-20. [Photograph] Retrieved from the Library of Congress,

https://www.loc.gov/item/2021756279/.

Historical Women. (3/18/2020) Retrieved from http://www.persepolis.nu/queens.htm

Hutyra, H. (2019). *123 Of the Most Powerful Martin Luther King Jr. Quotes Ever.* Retrieved

from https://www.keepinspiring.me/martin-luther-king-jr-quotes/#

Hutyra, H. (2019). 120 George Washington Quotes to Celebrate His Place in History

Retrieved from https://www.keepinspiring.me/george-washington-quotes/

Ideal Immigration. (2019). Retrieved from https://www.idealimmigration.us/blog/immigrants-in-
music

Isaacson, W. (2007). *Einstein: His Life and Universe.* Simon & Schuster.

Jang, M. (2017). Emma Watson, Beyoncé, 23 More Stars on Embracing Feminism and

Empowering Women. Retrieved from https://www.hollywoodreporter.com/lists/international-
womens-day-2017-feminist-quotes-25-celebrities-983702/item/uzo-aduba-international-
womens-day-2017-984410

Juma, N. (2020). Florence Nightingale quotes on Life, Communication and Nursing. Retrieved from https://everydaypower.com/florence-nightingale-quotes/

Kaivalya, A. (2016). *Myths of the Asanas: The Stories at the Heart of the Yoga Tradition*. Simon and Schuster.

Karen, H.C. (2015). *The Story of the Yoga Warrior Poses.* Retrieved from http://www.whenlifeisgood.com/the-story-of-the-yoga-warrior-poses/

Kendall, J., Waddington, C., and Kendall, C. (2005). The daily moment: a stress reduction program for cancer center staff. *J. Oncol. Manage.* 14, 68–71.

Kokugo Dai Jiten, 1988. Revised Edition. Retrieved from: https://en.wikipedia.org/wiki/Tokyo

Kripalu/School of Yoga. (2019). 200-Hour Teacher Training Manual.

Leffler, W. K., photographer. (1965) *Martin Luther King Press conf.* , 1965. March 2. [Photograph] Retrieved from the Library of Congress, https://www.loc.gov/item/2016646651/

Ludwig van Beethoven Quotes. (n.d.). BrainyQuote.com. Retrieved June 6, 2020, from BrainyQuote.com Web site: https://www.brainyquote.com/authors/ludwig-van-beethoven-quotes

Mayor, L. (2000, July 1). "Oprah: The Soul and Spirit of a Superstar: An Unofficial Tribute." *Amazon*, Triumph, 2000, www.amazon.com/Oprah-Winfrey-Soul-Spirit-Superstar/dp/1572434082.

Marie Curie Quotes. (n.d.). BrainyQuote.com. Retrieved June 6, 2020, from BrainyQuote.com Web site: https://www.brainyquote.com/authors/marie-curie-quotes

McGinley, K. (2017). *Uncover the Symbolism in 10 Common Yoga Poses.* Retrieved from https://chopra.com/articles/uncover-the-symbolism-in-10-common-yoga-poses

Neffe, J. (2007). *Einstein: A biography*. Farrar, Straus and Giroux. Retrieved from

https://books.google.com/books?hl=en&lr=&id=B8K6n177ZwcC&oi=fnd&pg=PR7&dq=Ein

stein+Biography+jurgen&ots=_trvRoc0hO&sig=9mWHvsJ-

ypQYNtQL4w5IUmEdjxY#v=onepage&q=Einstein%20Biography%20jurgen&f=false

Newsday.com Staff. (02/01/2017) Celebrities who are immigrants: Justin Bieber, Mila Kunis,

Pamela Anderson, more. Retrieved from

https://www.newsday.com/entertainment/celebrities/celebrities-who-are-immigrants-justin-

bieber-mila-kunis-pamela-anderson-more-1.5579736

Pennebaker, J. W., & Seagal, J. D. (1999). Forming a story: The health benefits of

narrative. *Journal of clinical psychology*, *55*(10), 1243-1254.

Reef, C. (2016). *Florence Nightingale: The Courageous Life of the Legendary

Nurse* (Illustrated). Clarion Books.

Radha, S. S. (2006). *Hatha yoga: the hidden language*. timeless books.

Savage, M. (2020). Coronavirus: Stars take part in One World: Together At Home concert. BBC

Music Composer. Retrieved from https://www.bbc.com/news/entertainment-arts-52333890

Sjoman, N. E. (1999). *The Yoga Tradition of the Mysore Palace* (2nd ed.). Abhinav Publications.

Thayer, A. W., & Krehbiel, H. E. (2020). *The Life of Ludwig van Beethoven (Vol. 1-3):

Complete Edition*. e-artnow.

Tillich, P. (2008). *The courage to be*. Yale University Press.

Trejo, N. (2019, June 10). *Angelina Jolie Has Made the World A Better Place, One Deed at A

Time*. Retrieved from https://us.hola.com/celebrities/gallery/2019061024598/angelina-jolie-

humanitGarcian-work-gallery/1/

Trikosko, M. S., photographer. (1979) *Interview with Cesar Chavez. 4/20/. Chavez gesturing.* ,
1979. [Photograph] Retrieved from the Library of Congress,
https://www.loc.gov/item/2016646413/

Turner, O. J., photographer. (ca. 1947) *Albert Einstein, -1955.*, ca. 1947. [Photograph] Retrieved
from the Library of Congress, https://www.loc.gov/item/2004671908/.

Weidenbach, A. & Stuart, G. (ca. 1876) *"George Washington" / A. Weidenbach.* , ca. 1876.
[1876] [Photograph] Retrieved from the Library of Congress,
https://www.loc.gov/item/2009633671/

Weisberger, M. (2017, June 2). *Beyond Wonder Woman: 12 Mighty Female Warriors.* Retrieved
from https://www.livescience.com/59330-beyond-wonder-women-real-female-warriors.html

Whittaker, Elizabeth; Robin M. Kowalski (2015). "Cyberbullying Via Social Media". *Journal of
School Violence*. 14 (1): 19. doi:10.1080/15388220.2014.949377. S2CID 144140856.

Wikipedia contributors. (2022, May 31). Albert Einstein. In *Wikipedia, The Free Encyclopedia.*
Retrieved 11:31, June 6, 2022,
from https://en.wikipedia.org/w/index.php?title=Albert_Einstein&oldid=960064108

Wikipedia contributors. (2022, June 6). Florence Nightingale. In *Wikipedia, The Free
Encyclopedia*. Retrieved 11:52, June 6, 2022,
from https://en.wikipedia.org/wiki/Florence_Nightingale

Wikipedia contributors. (2022, February 24). On the Floor. In *Wikipedia, The Free
Encyclopedia*. Retrieved 22:02, March 11, 2022,
from https://en.wikipedia.org/w/index.php?title=On_the_Floor&oldid=942426674

Wikipedia contributors. (2020, March 4). Pitbull (rapper). In *Wikipedia, The Free Encyclopedia*. Retrieved 22:00, March 11, 2020,

from https://en.wikipedia.org/w/index.php?title=Pitbull_(rapper)&oldid=943882623

Wikipedia contributors. (2022, June 6). Martin Luther King Jr. In *Wikipedia, The Free Encyclopedia*. Retrieved 11:05, June 6, 2022,

from https://en.wikipedia.org/w/index.php?title=Martin_Luther_King_Jr.&oldid=961007646

Wikipedia contributors. (2022, June 6). Ludwig van Beethoven. In *Wikipedia, The Free Encyclopedia*. Retrieved 11:17, June 6, 2022,

from https://en.wikipedia.org/w/index.php?title=Ludwig_van_Beethoven&oldid=961002658

Wikipedia contributors. (2022, June 3). Marie Curie. In *Wikipedia, The Free Encyclopedia*. Retrieved 11:40, June 6, 2022,

from https://en.wikipedia.org/w/index.php?title=Marie_Curie&oldid=960619663

Wikipedia contributors. (2020, June 20). COVID-19 pandemic. In *Wikipedia, The Free Encyclopedia*. Retrieved 19:56, June 20, 2020.

Wikipedia contributors. (2022, November). Hatshepsut. http://en.wikipedia.org/wiki/Hatshepsut